Crossing the Phantom Pass

Crossing the Phantom Pass

A Cancer Journey

Julia Kwong

Foreword by Arthur Kleinman

AEVO   **UNIVERSITY OF
TORONTO PRESS**

Aevo UTP
An imprint of University of Toronto Press
Toronto Buffalo London
utppublishing.com

Library and Archives Canada Cataloguing in Publication

Title: Crossing the phantom pass : a cancer journey / Julia Kwong ; foreword by Arthur Kleinman.
Names: Kwong, Julia, author | Kleinman, Arthur, writer of foreword
Description: Includes bibliographical references and index.
Identifiers: Canadiana (print) 20250176548 | Canadiana (ebook) 20250178885 | ISBN 9781487565916 (cloth) | ISBN 9781487565930 (EPUB) | ISBN 9781487565923 (PDF)
Subjects: LCSH: Kwong, Julia – Health. | LCSH: Kwong, Julia – Family. | LCSH: Breast – Cancer – Patients – Biography. | LCSH: Breast – Cancer – Treatment. | LCSH: Cancer – Patients – Family relationships. | LCSH: Fathers and daughters.
Classification: LCC RC280.B8 .K96 2025 | DDC 362.19699/4490092 – dc23

ISBN 978-1-4875-6591-6 (cloth)   ISBN 978-1-4875-6593-0 (EPUB)
                                     ISBN 978-1-4875-6592-3 (PDF)

Printed in Canada

Cover design: Heng Wee Tan
Cover image: iStock.com/HRAUN

We wish to acknowledge the land on which the University of Toronto Press operates. This land is the traditional territory of the Wendat, the Anishnaabeg, the Haudenosaunee, the Métis, and the Mississaugas of the Credit First Nation.

University of Toronto Press acknowledges the financial support of the Government of Canada, the Canada Council for the Arts, and the Ontario Arts Council, an agency of the Government of Ontario, for its publishing activities.

Canada Council   Conseil des Arts
for the Arts   du Canada

ONTARIO ARTS COUNCIL
CONSEIL DES ARTS DE L'ONTARIO
an Ontario government agency
un organisme du gouvernement de l'Ontario

Funded by the   Financé par le
Government   gouvernement
of Canada   du Canada

Canada

MIX
Paper | Supporting
responsible forestry
FSC
www.fsc.org   FSC® C103567

Contents

Foreword by Arthur Kleinman   vii

Disclaimer   xii

1 You've Got Cancer   1

2 A Tough Decision   17

3 Getting Past Gatekeepers   33

4 Outward Calm   49

5 Excision   63

6 Fatigue   79

7 Culinary Advice, Friendly Support   89

8 Bills to Pay   105

9 Radiation   117

10 Shopping Aerobics   129

11 Weekend of Anguish   139

12 Lost   149

13 Days of Hell   165

14 Grasping for Help   177

15 Safe at Last   189

16 Another Lifeline   201

17 Home Again   217

18 Epilogue   227

Bibliography   237

Index   239

Foreword

What happens when a social scientist, skilled in applying social theoretical models to everyday social institutions, relationships, and experiences, learns from her doctor that she has cancer? Unsurprisingly, the academic distance drops away, as does the methodological quest for "objectivity" and "generalizability." Knowledge of Talcott Parsons's famous model of the sick role seems almost beside the point. Fear, anger, disorientation, the anxious uncertainty of constrained hope – all undermine intellectualization as a personal coping style and professional persona. The existential threat dissolves competence and confidence. It requires courage and endurance. The medical regimen – so readily available to criticize when experienced as a distant, impersonal framing of the problems of others – is embraced as a lifeline with potential to make one a survivor. And the serious illness experience and simultaneous disablement of a distant elderly parent parallels the acute distress of one's cancer care, creating high tension between balancing self-care and family care.

Professor Julia Kwong's cancer narrative takes up the story from here, emphasizing a middle-aged Chinese North American cancer patient's many meetings with the various doctors and nurses who will care for her over the years of her troubled quest for cure and palliation. Along the way, Professor Kwong experienced what many of us have experienced with our chaotic, broken healthcare system: delays, miscommunications, insensitive treatment, frustrating attitudes, bias, and both the lack of warmth and emotional support and its opposite. The doctors she encounters in a smaller second-tier city range from the careless to the careful, from those who have embraced the moral and emotional responsibilities of their work to those who seem preoccupied by the power of institutional efficiency to make quality care seem an impossible dream and to substitute for that dream a selfish focus on generating income while practicing without the warmth of real presence.

Because she is Chinese, Professor Kwong's experiences regularly raise cultural questions that inflect the economic and social concerns she has had to juggle. Because she is a woman, again not surprisingly, the family care she receives is less developed than the family care she provides for her father and herself. And because she is in a small city, there is no cancer care team to integrate different specialized skills into a dependable holistic system. The neoliberal government is present through the absence of an adequate local healthcare system.

The lived experience of the quest for care for cancer in this personal account is an authentic contribution to the literature of personal memoirs of serious illness and exacting treatment that is democratizing healthcare. Patient voices and the experience of family carers have never before been so available and insistent, there illustrating not just the complexity of care, but its limits, failures, and resurgence. Care is among those things that matter most in our lives. Yet what characterizes care today is the enormous burden on the sick and their families, who must become the integrators and sustainers of caregiving. Here kinship relationships, such as spousal ties and the quality of interactions between adult children and their elderly parents, do most of the behind-the-scenes work of care. Much of this remains invisible to health professionals. Yet it is crucial to survival, improvement, palliation, and the management of death and dying.

Our world has become bureaucratized to a degree that would have even surprised Max Weber, the supreme sociological analyst of early twentieth-century bureaucratic rationality and institutional efficiency. Taken together with big business and big government, this behemoth dominates the medical landscape of hospitals, clinics, pharmacies, and insurance companies. The saddening outcome is the loss of professional autonomy and the weakening of patient and family control over care. Doctors today are employees, workers on the shop floor of ever-expanding healthcare institutional systems. And yet they still struggle to provide quality care that is personal and technical. What we have learned over half a century is that patients and families constitute the very center of health-care decision-making, actions, and evaluations of out-come. Nonetheless, they do not have formal control over the levers of power in each of these areas. It is the informal network-based heart of healthcare that experiences and copes with suffering, its financial and psychological burdens, and the difficulties of treatment and rehabilitation. But these informal networks do not have the legitimacy to negotiate the complexities and intricacies of the healthcare system. However, it is these same lay or popular circles of care that bring moral and humanistic concerns into the mundane work of caregiving and into the struggles that medical professionals experience in attempting to understand and engage these humanistic processes. Patients, doctors, nurses, and families are the human beings at the core of care. Even a sea of regulations and capitalist profit-making cannot eliminate this basic human element. But it can make it look, feel, and actually be very different in the 2020s than in the 1950s and '60s.

This book is good to think with. The experiences it describes are a sample of the vast variety of human experiences of cancer and cancer care. Each human experience in itself carries the choke and sting of a particular person's personal pain as well as their frustrations with care and care giving. Each experience illustrates the dangers and uncertainties of our lives as patients, family carers, and professional healers. Each experience brings history and context into confrontation with therapeutic algorithms. Each experience requires of us a passion for care and caregiving in order to endure the institutional systems that dominate healthcare. And each experience shows why care still really matters.

Arthur Kleinman, MD, is Professor of Medical Anthropology, Global Health and Social Medicine, and Psychiatry at Harvard University, and the author of *The Soul of Care*.

Disclaimer

This memoir is a personal account of the author's experiences as a patient. Names, locations, and identifying characteristics have been changed to protect privacy. The reflections and opinions shared are solely those of the author; they are not intended as medical advice. Readers should consult qualified healthcare professionals for any medical concerns.

ONE

You've Got Cancer

"You've got cancer," Dr. Chang said.

Complete silence followed; no one said a word. In the stillness I distinguished three voices in the next room. I could not make out what they were saying, but the tone suggested they were talking about something serious – something to be expected in an examination room in a hospital outpatient clinic. Most probably a doctor, a patient, and a companion were discussing a medical problem and treatment. This was my guess.

People feel uncomfortable when no words are exchanged. When one person says something, another in the room is expected to respond; when this does not happen, even the speaker sometimes may feel obliged to say something, anything, to break the ice. This is social expectation. Dr. Chang felt the pressure; to fill the void he expanded on his earlier statement.

"You need surgery. If you do not remove it, you will have about two years to live."

If the doctor thought his words would elicit a response, he was wrong. His elaboration of the earlier prognosis only solidified the silence. A "death sentence" or perhaps the "life sentence" from a doctor will stun any recipient; even other listeners around may not know what to say. No one said a word and the silence resumed. Once more the muffled conversation of the three voices in the next room became audible. I did not know how long the eavesdropping lasted.

"You have no use of it. You might as well have it out." These words broke the silence; they came from me.

The pronouncement of impending doom was meant for my father; the "it" was his prostate. We were in the urology department of Youde Hospital, a public hospital named after a former British governor in Hong Kong. Almost twenty years after China took the colony back from the British in 1997, much of the dual-track public/private healthcare system the British put in place remained. Like many Hong Kong citizens, Father was using the much-subsidized public healthcare system with facilities and doctors as good if not better than most private ones.

For more than a year, Father found blood in his urine. A government doctor examined him, diagnosed it as a bladder infection, and prescribed Cipro. The bleeding stopped for a while and returned; the search for the cause of the problem started again. Father saw more than one doctor and more than a few times; even a microscopic camera up the urethra all the way to the kidneys found nothing out of the ordinary. Only a moment ago did the doctor come up with the answer: my father had late-stage prostate cancer.

I lived across the Pacific 7,000 miles away from Hong Kong and happened to be visiting my father on the day of his medical appointment. I met Dr. Chang for the first time, and I believed for Father too. As a patient using the public healthcare system, Father did not have one doctor following his case; he saw different ones depending on who was on duty the day of the appointment. The attending doctor on the occasion, however, was always on top of his case because his medical file was kept in a centralized data bank together with that of other patients using the public healthcare system and was accessible to government doctors.

I did not know what Dr. Chang made of my remark, "You have no use of it." Father looked young for someone in his late eighties, trim and fit with few wrinkles on his forehead; his bald crown framed by a narrow crescent of thinning gray hair only added an aura of respectability not years to his looks. In contrast, I could be taken for someone beyond my sixties. My hair had turned gray, my lips thinned, and my cheeks hollowed. When we were out together people often took me for his partner; the doctor probably thought the same, especially after what I said. I was the outspoken if not the shameless disgruntled wife of a sexually impotent old man. Dr. Chang could think what he wanted; it did not matter to me. I did not care, and I was not in the mood to clarify the relationship. I had a more important problem to think about.

I sat a little behind Father across the doctor stationed behind his big, imposing desk in the narrow examination room. I could not see my father's face. He sat perfectly motionless, not a single muscle twitching on his back; most likely he looked equally impassive in the front, and he did not utter a single word.

The doctor was taken aback by the patient's lack of response and turned to me.

"Does he understand Chinese?" he asked.

What was this doctor thinking? To ask another in Chinese if this Chinese-looking, Chinese-speaking person sitting in front of him spoke Chinese! Father taught me the language!

"He does," I answered.

Again, Father sat perfectly still, not a word escaped from his lips.

The doctor and I discussed treatment – the surgery, its benefits and risks, and how long the patient would take to recuperate. Arrangements were made for the operation; surgery was to take place in three weeks, and Father signed the consent form without saying a word.

Father had a catheter put in while waiting for the operation. He developed an infection two weeks later, something not exactly unusual for someone with the insert. He was hospitalized. After being bed-ridden for a week, he developed a blood clot in his left leg and was put on blood thinners. The drug proved a little too strong and he bled internally. Needless to say, the series of complications caused delay. Father became too weak for the operation and never received it.

But Father proved the doctor wrong; he beat the odds. The two years Dr. Chang gave him came and went. He might not always feel good, but he remained active, going out to restaurants, going to the movies, going to the park, and going to wherever, whenever, with whomever invited him. He did well for a ninety-year-old, especially for someone with his medical condition.

A man of this age would not live forever even without a diagnosis of terminal prostate cancer. After the meeting with Dr. Chang I became very conscious of Father's mortality and made a point to fly across the Pacific to see him at least once a year, sometimes more than once if the situation required. I would be back if Father took a turn for the worse and had to be hospitalized, but he made it out of the hospital every time. I kept the same routine this year, bought a ticket for the sixteen-hour direct flight from Los Angeles to Hong Kong.

I took the medical profession's recommendation and usually had a mammogram done before my annual flying ritual. This year was no different. I scheduled the screening two weeks before I was to leave. A couple of days after taking the mammogram someone at the family doctor's office called.

"I am calling from Dr. Gray's office. You have to go for a mammogram again."

Dr. Gray is a pseudonym and indeed the names of all the doctors and healthcare professionals to be mentioned in these pages. This is to protect their identities. I was puzzled by the request and said nothing. The caller noticed the hesitation and explained.

"The film is not clear; you need to do it again. You can do it tomorrow. Can you make it?"

Her explanation sounded plausible; I believed her. A glitch in the machine; I had to do it again to get a clearer picture. She did not exactly say that, that was what I had thought. I am not the worrying type and did not give the call too much thought. Moreover, experience is a great teacher. I had had lumps in my breasts before, once in my twenties and again in my forties; they turned out to be benign both times. These earlier encounters gave me confidence that everything would be all right. Taking out the cysts, tumors, nodules, or whatever the medical profession may call these lumps can be painful. The first time for more than two weeks I felt pain with every movement of the body after the operation; even slow walking sent jitters to the incision. Perhaps practice made perfect even for the patient, though more than likely medical techniques had improved in the intervening years. The second time the pain was not so bad and the discomfort went away in a little more than a week. If I had to go through the procedure one more time, with such experiences behind me the operation would be a walk in the park.

The caller phoned again the day following the second mammography, or it could have been a different person. This time she asked me to go in for a sonogram, more commonly known as an ultrasound. This was something new. I had two operations to remove breast tumors, but I never had an ultrasound. I was a little puzzled but still not worried.

Mammography takes pictures of tissues with X-rays; sonography's high-frequency sound waves can tell a cyst from a tumor. I had friends who had undergone one or the other procedure, and those who had taken both all agreed that getting an ultrasound brings less discomfort without the two panels pressing on the breast in mammography. The assurance of less discomfort was good but meant little to me; I am a stoic – if I have to do something, I will go through with it regardless.

The stoicism had something to do with my upbringing. I grew up in the British colony of Hong Kong after the Second World War; the place was not the booming, bustling city of today. Life was difficult. Our family shipping supply business came to a halt when the war started and ships stopped calling. With no income coming in, Grandfather turned to the family coffer. Family is very important for the Chinese, and more so many decades ago. To feed his immediate family, the extended one, and any relative who came knocking on the door, Grandfather sold one property after another. Four years later, when the war was over, we were paying rent for the house we once owned. If I complained of hardships growing up, my parents would remind me that my challenges were nothing compared to what they went through during those tumultuous war years. They told stories of the sudden Japanese air raids, fleeing from the house at short notice, ducking into bomb shelters, and some returning only to find their homes flattened. They also told stories of people rummaging through the garbage for any leftover food only to find nothing, and some swallowing human hair to ease their hunger only to die as a consequence. Their descriptions of the emaciated corpses found on the street in the early hours of the morning before the authorities could take them away gave me nightmares. I was told to stop whining, work hard, be strong, and to take on the challenges coming my way.

Being a girl, I was also told to be cool not in the current sense of being culturally "with it," but to act "proper." I was to be demure and gentle, displaying behavior becoming to the weaker sex, a positive rather than derogatory term at the time, and feminine traits that would be condemned these days. My parents were to be sadly disappointed because I turned out to be far from feminine or docile. I was the tomboy playing rough and tumble with my two brothers, even wrestling with them on the floor. With enough repetition, however, some of my parents' teaching did seep in. I may not be the lady they had hoped for, but I am even keel, not easily excitable, not effusive in expressing my emotions, and reticent to articulate my opinions.

I did not lose any sleep over the weekend. Nine o'clock the following Monday I was at the clinic where I had taken the mammogram, only this time it was for the sonogram. I was ushered into a small room with a bed and the usual paraphernalia of impressive if not imposing medical equipment. Next to the bed was a light grayish metal console on wheels with a host of knobs, switches, and wiring attached to the casing and a TV monitor perched on top. I was too ignorant to comprehend its function or to be impressed by this gadget of advanced technology.

I lay on the bed stripped to the waist. A woman employee – or to be more specific, the diagnostic imaging technician or ultrasonographer – applied gel on my right breast and moved the transducer, a hand-held club-like instrument attached to the machine, back and forth over it. As if she had found something, she zeroed in on the spot to the left of the nipple, crisscrossing the area several times; my untrained eyes glued to the screen saw only wavy lines and blurry bubbles emerging and receding reminding me of pictures of the uterus of a pregnant woman I saw on television. I did not know what to make of what I saw. Now I know. She was looking for the tumor and found it; I only saw wriggles on the black-and-white screen.

Two days later I was back in the same room with the same technician to harvest breast tissues for biopsy. A woman in a doctor's white coat walked into the room. She had black hair, high cheekbones, dark brown almond-shaped eyes, a delicately bridged nose, a small mouth, and skin the same color as mine. She had to be Chinese. On another occasion I would have asked if she was and if she answered in the affirmative, I would inquire if she spoke Chinese; and if she did, I would speak to her in my native language. Even after living in America for forty years, I like to converse in my mother tongue and have never missed an opportunity to do so when the occasion comes. Speaking the language in Chinese restaurants in small towns always got me better service from the waiter, special attention from the chef, larger food servings than the other customers, and perhaps free deserts; sometimes it worked even in big-city restaurants. I was not sure what perks I would get from a doctor in a medical office if I did the same.

The repeated breast examinations had to have rattled me because I did not attempt to strike up a conversation in Chinese even when I suspected the doctor was of my same ethnicity. The ultrasonographer told me afterward that the doctor was Chinese and spoke Cantonese, my local dialect. I missed my chance. The Chinese doctor explained in English that she would numb the breast with localized anesthesia and then obtain a specimen from the nodule for biopsy. She gave me a shot of anesthetic and waited for the drug to take effect; it didn't take long. The technician located the tumor with the hammerhead transducer in no time, and the doctor punctured my skin with a long needle attached to a syringe. Instead of giving me an injection, she used the syringe like a vacuum cleaner to suck tissue samples from the breast.

After the aspiration procedure, the doctor explained that she would go in from another side to tag the nodule to facilitate locating it in the future. The dirty word "cancer" was never uttered, but reality was closing in. My thoughts were racing.

"Stapling the tumor to find it another time? They are not finished with me. There is more to come. I have to come back again? That doesn't sound right." It did not occur to me the next stop might not be the clinic but a hospital. These questions whirled in my head, and I was too preoccupied with my thoughts to monitor what the doctor was doing. The procedure was finished before I knew it; I had another mammogram to make sure the marker stayed in place.

The ultrasound-guided biopsy took place at ten in the morning, and I was barely home after meeting a friend for lunch when someone from Dr. Gray's office called asking me to go in the next day. Getting a medical appointment is never easy and almost impossible to have one at short notice if I had wanted it; an offer to see me first thing in the morning without my asking? The doctor was treating the matter too seriously for my comfort. I often tell friends who are impatient to find out the results of medical tests that no news is good news; when the medical profession takes the initiative to contact a patient, something may be wrong. These are not just comforting words for friends; I do believe this to be the case. The alacrity with which Dr. Gray was handling my case told me something was not right.

"What's it about?" I asked when the caller offered me the next-day appointment.

"I don't know." The should-be-expected standard answer from trained medical personnel.

"Has the biopsy report come in? What did it say?"

"I don't know. I do not have it. You have to ask the doctor." Another standard to-be-expected response. No medical staff in their right minds would answer questions like these over the phone. I should have known better than to ask, but I could not stop myself.

Victor, my husband, was the worrying type; I had not mentioned to him my repeated visits to the diagnostic clinic. That evening I told him about the next-day medical appointment; he was with me when Dr. Gray walked into the examination room.

Dr. Gray has been our family doctor for as long as we have been living in this sun-belt city. He majored in physics in his undergraduate years, and Victor, a retired physicist, picked him as the family doctor for this and no other reason. Most friends thought physics was a difficult subject and physicists were intelligent; Victor thought so, and so did Dr. Gray. The doctor exuded the self-confidence of a physicist if not that of the medical doctor, or more than likely both.

"We're about the same age," I said one time. We were one year apart.

"I have more experience," he corrected me. The message was clear; I was not in his league.

We, and it was really Victor and the doctor, became friendly over the years. On our nothing-more-than-routine checkups every six months, the two would talk about new discoveries and recent scientific breakthroughs before going into what we came for – shining the otoscope into the ear canal, holding down the tongue with a depressor to peer at the tonsils, a few taps on the back, and listening to the stethoscope bell resting against the chest. They spent more time chatting about science than the doctor spent performing these routines on the two patients.

The doctor came in wearing his standard knee-length white coat over light-blue shirt and dark pants. He never wore a tie. He shook hands with me perched on the examination table and then with Victor sitting in the chair. No small talk and nothing on science. He approached the counter with the thick file of my medical records the nurse had pulled a little earlier. Despite his science background he had not moved into the computer age and his patient records were still in pen and ink. He looked at a page in the file and said these words without turning his head.

"You've got cancer."

Opening the file, turning the pages, and reading from it were merely props, preamble to the announcement he was to make; he knew all along what he had to say before he crossed the threshold.

The term "cancer" comes from the Greek word for crab. Hippocrates, the father of medicine, called cancer "crab" or "karkinos" because the tumor, with its veins extending outward, reminded him of the crustacean. The name seems most appropriate to me for a different reason. Cancer, like a crab, grips the patient with its strong hard claws, gives the person great discomfort and suffering, and sometimes never lets go. To be diagnosed with cancer is frightening; the person knows it is serious only he does not know how "serious" the problem is or what lies ahead. There is usually waiting with more tests to follow, leaving the patient in limbo and anxious to know what is in store. Then there is the preparation for the treatment, and then the treatment. The treatment procedure can take weeks and sometimes months, and it can come with side effects not always easy to take. When the treatment phase is over and the cancer is in remission, the patient is left with the fear of the malignant cells resurfacing, migrating, and infecting other organs. Metastasis is the frightful medical term for the spread of cancer.

Father was going through that with his prostate cancer. With the operation abandoned some six years ago because of the infection, blood clot, and internal bleeding, he took Casodex to halt cancer growth. The drug was effective for a couple of years and then stopped working. Cancer spread to his spine and he had difficulty walking. Palliative radiation on the spine gave him some mobility; then his belly became distended and he was in constant discomfort. He told his children he did not want any more intrusive medical intervention. My two brothers and I agreed that treatment would only bring our father discomfort and might not help; we went along with his wishes. We let it go and since then we did not attempt to find out how far or how much the cancer had spread.

Earlier in the year my brother, a doctor, said our father had perhaps about a year to live. He was right on when he made a similar prediction on our mother's imminent passing eight years ago; I trusted his prognosis and all the more wanted to see Father with his end closing in. A plane ticket was purchased, my bags were packed, and a bed was waiting in my father's apartment for my arrival the following Wednesday. Dr. Gray's pronouncement did not come as a complete surprise in the wake of the repeated tests and examinations. They probably prepared me for the news. In fact, the words sounded strangely familiar. I heard almost the same words in the urology clinic in Hong Kong six years ago, only it was said in Chinese and meant for Father; now the message was in English and meant for me. Having heard those words once before should not have expurgated fear, especially when I was the recipient of the bad news. Strange enough, I was not fearful. No alarm bells rang; I did not feel anything different.

What came out of my mouth was as spontaneous and natural as my breathing.

"I am leaving for Hong Kong on Monday," I said matter-of-factly. I would be going to see my father in a couple of days.

Looking back, the response was a surprise even to me. Was I telling the doctor I had something better to do and no time for treatment? Was I saying I would do nothing about the cancer? Did I not recognize the gravity of the situation? I had to know that breast cancer was a disease serious enough to warrant doing something about as soon as possible. What did I mean? My reaction did not make sense.

My eyes were fixed on Dr. Gray's salt-and-pepper head of hair bent over the file. As he slowly turned his head to face me, our eyes met. I looked straight at him and did not blink; he returned my cold stare with an equally dispassionate gaze. We were mirror images of each other – the doctor as cold and inscrutable as the patient perched on the examination table across from him. We were cowboys locked in a duel, staring each other down to see who would blink first; only we were not about to draw our guns to kill.

The doctor did not appear surprised or offended by my ridiculous if not irrational outburst; if he was, he did not show it. Perhaps he was right; he had seen a lot and had more life experience than me. He was not floored by my reaction. Instead, he dispensed the following advice with a solemn expression on his face and in a tone becoming a medical practitioner addressing a patient on a serious medical problem.

"Medical treatment there should be similar. You can have the surgery in Hong Kong and complete the radiation here."

He knew my annual visits to see Father in Hong Kong and he had offered me a way out; he gave me an action plan in not so many words. I would have the tumor removed in Hong Kong and recover from the operation before coming back for further treatment. This would provide me some time to spend with Father.

I did not utter a word of response, but my eyes softened and the muscles on my face relaxed to signal acceptance of his proposal. Dr. Gray got the message. He closed the file on the counter and was about to walk out of the room.

"I need a copy of the biopsy report." At least I had the wits to ask.

"The office will give you a copy," the doctor answered without turning his head and closed the door behind him.

The meeting could not have lasted more than ten minutes, and it might have been shorter. The doctor told me I had cancer and did not identify the location; I knew it was in the breast without his saying. I told him I would be going to Hong Kong; he knew I was going to see Father and did not persuade me to do anything different. We did not say much, but we said enough to understand each other; there was a problem and the doctor came up with the solution to break the impasse. He offered me a compromise treatment plan.

The conversation was succinct; it was between the doctor and me. Victor did not say a word. This pattern of exchange would continue in all subsequent medical appointments – Victor would be present but mute at every meeting. An eavesdropper in the next room would never suspect a third person was there. Knowing him, I knew Victor would be listening intently, analyzing everything said, busily deliberating what to do next, and fearful of the worst. Months later when I asked how he felt at this initial meeting, I got a rhetorical answer – "You don't think I could have been happy?" The rest was for me to fill in.

We walked to the front entrance of Dr. Gray's office, now the exit. Six patients sat waiting in the lobby; no one looked up when we passed. If someone did, the person could not and would not have guessed the life-changing news we just heard. One of us could have just been diagnosed with the flu and gotten a prescription from the doctor; we did not look any different. But our lives were forever changed.

TWO

A Tough Decision

A tumor is not made in a day; mine had to have been there for some time. In the last couple of years Father's health was failing and I worried. It seemed I was constantly on the go, visiting Hong Kong at least once a year and sometimes on short notice, like that time I dropped everything to go when he suddenly took a turn for the worse and went into intensive care. The frequent travels probably took a toll on me, or perhaps the stress of worrying about him did.

My health had not been great. My body lost its internal thermostat and had difficulty adjusting to the slightest temperature change. I had leg cramps when the temperature dropped a few degrees and sweated profusely when the weather warmed up. Acid reflux woke me up in the middle of the night, and I took warm milk heated in the microwave to soothe my stomach before I could return to sleep. I have always been allergic to pollen and dust and reacted more strongly to these allergens. My nose was stuffed and I had to prop three pillows under my head before I felt comfortable enough to sleep at night. I stayed indoors as much as possible in spring – alas, the best time of the year to be outside! In the morning, my eyes were glued shut with sticky discharge from conjunctivitis; I had to rinse them under a running tap to get rid of the grit and gunk before I could see. The worst was the persistent cough that again kept me from having a good night's rest. I took every brand of cough syrup to no avail until a doctor in Chinese medicine prescribed an herbal concoction from his personal pharmacy on one of my Hong Kong visits. I boiled what he gave me, drank it, and the cough went away without me ever knowing what I took. I blamed these problems on the stress from worrying about Father and on age. Now that I knew I had cancer, I could not help wondering if these were symptoms of cancer weakening the body and lowering the immune system, or perhaps cancer was just another by-product of the stress I had been going through.

I might not feel anything different when Dr. Gray said, "You've got cancer"; with those words I became a bona fide cancer patient. I did not know how cancer patients should feel or react or how they usually felt or reacted on hearing the news; I thought I should feel something, something different, with the cataclysmic news. But I did not. I was not taken by surprise; the repeated tests might have prepared me for it. Neither did I know what I was thinking or if I was thinking. It almost seemed news of my breast cancer was something I heard over the radio with little or nothing to do with me.

I was puzzled with the reaction. When I mentioned it to a social worker friend, she explained my lack of reaction as one of those body defenses to extreme threats or catastrophes. She could be right. I might not have been exposed to the bomb explosions, mutilated body parts, or the other goriness of war that soldiers faced on the battlefield, but I could be shell-shocked just the same. I was stunned; my insistence on going to Hong Kong might be a sign of the trauma. I was shocked to fully appreciate the gravity of the situation.

I could think of a few other possible explanations too. The numbness could be denial, not wanting to believe I had cancer and not wanting to think about what to do about it. Sticking to the travel schedule might have been this kind of reaction. Or it could be an indication of my inflexibility, slow to adjust to changing circumstances. If it was the latter case, I was the car with the ignition on, engine revving, going nowhere; or worse, heading straight on a disastrous course, and this would be dangerous. Looking back and knowing how things had developed, I was perhaps doing just that.

I spent thirty years working as a sociologist reading books, scouring through archives, and interviewing strangers I had never met before. I interviewed government officials in America and China; approached community leaders, long-time residents and new immigrants in the ethnic community; and talked to teachers and students in schools. I lectured to big and small classes of students, chaired seminars, and hosted meetings. I spoke in front of small and large audiences at academic conferences and public gatherings. Yet all the training and work experience failed me in the doctor's office. I did not ask Dr. Gray any questions about cancer or treatment; it did not occur to me to do so. Perhaps even if I had thought about doing it, I would not have known what questions to ask; I had to know something to ask something, and I did not know anything about breast cancer. I would not know where to start.

I might know something about prostate cancer trying to understand what was happening to Father in the last few years, but I knew nothing about my own kind of cancer. I only knew breast cancer was not something to be trifled with and could kill. A student who later became a close friend diagnosed with an aggressive breast cancer passed away two months before my visit to Dr. Gray's office.

Once home, my training and habituation to research kicked in, and I turned on the computer to get information on breast cancer. I googled the search term "breast cancer," and numerous websites came up. I knew to ignore the commercial sites of for-profit healthcare providers or pharmaceutical companies hawking their wares and zeroed in on those posted by reputable professional nonprofit organizations. I consulted those of the Mayo Clinic, the American Cancer Society, the Cancer Research Institute, and other such associations in the United States, United Kingdom, and Canada. I studied information provided by reputable medical schools and universities like Stanford, Johns Hopkins, Harvard, Yale, and others. In the months to follow I read books such as S. Mukerjhee's *Emperor of All Maladies*, Dr. Susan Love's *Breast Book*, the Mayo Clinic *Breast Cancer Book*, and other references. That day I only consulted the internet.

Cancer is the unchecked growth of normal cells that have mutated and changed their genetic structure. There is breast cancer, lung cancer, liver cancer, and indeed as many types of cancer as there are body parts, and these can be further categorized by the cancer's location within the organ. For example, breast cancer can be ductal or lobular, depending on where these cells nest in the breast. These abnormal cells have different structures and different characteristics; they can be invasive or noninvasive, benign or malignant, with some more lethal than others. There are three main types of breast cancer cells – estrogen receptor positive, progesterone receptor positive, and HER2 positive; the first two types of breast cancer cells bind with the hormones estrogen and progesterone to grow, and the last one flourishes in the presence of the protein HER2. Breast cancer is not all the same. Each person's cancer is a little different with a different combination or permutation of these malignant cells. Progression in cancer is measured in stages, with stage 4 being the most advanced. In breast cancer there is a stage 0, the pre-cancerous stage requiring only excision to get rid of the unwanted tumor. Staging is determined by the tumor size, location, nature of the cells, and more importantly, how far the unwanted cells have spread from the primary site.

The American Cancer Society has estimated that one in eight women will get breast cancer in their lifetime, and about 300,000 women are diagnosed with the disease every year. The rate is similar in Canada, with 30,000 diagnosed in a population one-tenth of that in the United States. Cancer occurs when healthy cells mutate; since cells are more likely to do that as a person gets older, the probability of getting breast cancer increases with age. On the flip side, these cells usually grow more slowly as one ages – a consoling thought for this senior diagnosed with the disease. Nevertheless, these research studies would suggest the number of breast cancer cases will rise with an aging population.

The good news is the breast cancer lobby is strong and long has the support of powerful and very visible women like Betty Ford. They were successful in soliciting funding for research; both the understanding and treatment of the disease have greatly improved over the years. The lobby has also been successful in introducing policies for screening. In Canada the government offers free breast checkups, and in the United States insurance companies cover annual mammogram screening. As a result, women find out early if they have breast cancer; when the disease is detected, early treatment is usually successful. It is said that if a person is to have cancer (and nobody wants that), breast cancer is supposedly the "best."

Cancer treatments have broadened from surgery, radiation, and chemotherapy to include target therapy and immunotherapy. Treatment may include one or more of these methods in any order tailored to the location, stage, type of cancer, as well as the health condition of the recipient. Surgery to take out the tumor is usually the first line of defense; when the tumor is large sometimes chemotherapy or radiation may be used to shrink it before taking it out. The surgical procedure serves both therapeutic and diagnostic purposes to take out the tumor and to determine the stage of the disease. Radiation uses high-energy rays to kill cancer cells in a circumscribed area, and chemotherapy is the infusion of a combination of different toxic chemicals to attack the cancer cells and almost inevitably affect the normal ones as well. It is known to result in hair loss, nausea, dry itchy skin, damaged nerves, and other unwanted side effects. Target therapy is an improvement over the shot gun approach of chemotherapy; the concoction aims only at the cancer cells, reducing the collateral damage on other tissues. And immunotherapy triggers the person's own defense system to fight these abnormal cells. The last two ways of treatment is an improvement over chemotherapy but comes with some deleterious side effects as well.

The successful treatment of cancer is measured by a person living five years "cancer free" after the initial diagnosis. To be "cancer free" may not mean the person carries no cancer cells in the body; it only means these cells are undetectable and not numerous enough to do harm. The medical establishment uses the term "in remission" when cancer is not detected, perhaps to highlight the possibility that cancer cells may still be there lurking inside to do harm at a later time. To reduce this probability, the person may receive adjuvant therapy, that is, taking drugs after the primary or active treatment phase to stave off the chance of cancer coming back.

I did not have this overall knowledge of cancer after I searched the web on the day of the diagnosis; I pieced this together over the course of treatment and after. At the time I was more interested in making sense of the information in the biopsy report in hand. The report labeled the cancer invasive ductal carcinoma and gave the location, type, size, and scores on numerous indicators with esoteric names. After the computer search, I did not know too much more; I did not understand what mitotic, tubular, or other scores meant, and even now I do not have any better of an idea. Nonetheless, as one lacking imagination or perhaps as an eternal optimist, I believed that the low scores on these indicators suggested I would not die from cancer, at least not in the near future. A person sometimes picks information to fit into what she wants to believe; I am no different. I clutched onto the information that bolstered what I wanted to be the case. I took the low scores on the indices to mean that my breast cancer was not serious, and I was reluctant to believe anything otherwise when indeed a low score might not necessarily be a good one; it might be the exact opposite. And I did not know the range of the score to know what the number meant; a score of three out of four would be very different from a three on a ten-point scale. I clung onto Dr. Gray's treatment plan for support. The web suggested that surgery and radiation were procedures reserved for those with early stages of the disease; Dr. Gray's game plan would put my cancer at stage 1 or at most stage 2. According to the American Cancer Society, the breast cancer survival rate of those with stage 1 cancer was cited as a 100 per cent and for those in stage 2, 93 per cent. I should have at least five years, if not more, to live.

I sat glued in front of the computer screen for hours frantically searching for information on breast cancer and treatment, cross-checking what I got from one website with those on others, and printed reams and reams of materials from the computer for future reference. I did not know where Victor was or what he was doing all that time. Neither can I remember if I cooked or ate at all. I was encased in my own world, searching for information on cancer and treatment oblivious of everything else.

I had been on the computer since late morning. It was past midnight before I stopped to think where the information would take me and to deliberate on the next course of action. Father expected me to be in Hong Kong next week; I could not delay departure unless I told him about the diagnosis. News of my cancer would add to his pain. He might not be able to take the news in his condition, and the knowledge might hasten his passing. I did not want to be the person to bring this possibility closer; I could not tell him. Moreover, I wanted to see him and to be with him in his remaining days. I might not be thinking clearly in the doctor's office, but this consideration might have been at the back of my mind to prompt me to say what I said – to leave for Hong Kong the following week regardless. Now that the doctor had given me his treatment plan and his blessing to go, the questions became how and where would I get surgery in Hong Kong?

The Hong Kong Breast Cancer Foundation reported the lifetime risk of women getting breast cancer as one in sixteen, half of the one in eight statistics given by Breastcancer. org in the United States. Even with this lower incidence rate in Hong Kong, it was not hard to find breast cancer "survivors" or women who once had breast cancer; two friends and a cousin had it some years ago.

Ever since I got cancer I had disliked the term "cancer survivor" and avoided using it as much as possible. The word "survivor" suggests the person has been near death; not everyone recovering from cancer has a close call; I did not. Some illnesses such as pneumonia can bring patients to the brink of demise, and we don't call those coming out of their ordeal survivors. Neither do I like the term "remission" even if a person entertains a chance of cancer coming back. There are other diseases that come back after a person recovers; a good example is shingles. A child recovers from chicken pox, but the virus may become active to give the person shingles later in life. My friends and I who grew up in Hong Kong had chicken pox when we were young; a few suffered from shingles in their senior years and their "small pox" was not labeled "in remission" in the interlude. I prefer to see cancer like any other illness – one develops a condition and is "cured" even though there is a possibility it may come back. Is my position avoidance? Cowardice? Eternal optimism? Stoicism? Or just pickiness on semantics? I don't know.

It was in the wee hours of the morning in North America and late afternoon in Hong Kong before I turned to the logistics of treatment. I called my friend Mary. She was not home; I tried her cell phone.

"Is it a good time to talk?"

I might have asked the question, but I had no intention to follow up with what I was supposed to do if her answer was a "no." I never called Mary on her cell phone, or "mobile" as it was called in Hong Kong, and I could hear the surprise in her voice. She told me she was in Wing On department store looking for a purse. It was of course not a good time to talk; her answer might as well be a no. She was too polite to say so and I was too anxious to wait to call another time. I proceeded to do what I started out to do.

"I have breast cancer and I am thinking of coming back for treatment." I explained; then I went directly to the point.

"You had it a couple of years ago, right?"

"What did you do? What treatment did you get?" I was direct and to the point.

"I had surgery, and then radiation." Great, just the treatment procedures Dr. Gray mentioned.

I followed with questions first on surgery, then on radiation.

"Where did you get the treatment?"

"Which hospital?"

"To whom did you go?"

"What's the surgeon's name?"

"How could I get hold of the doctor?"

"Any wait?"

"How long?"

"How long did the procedure take?"

"How many days were you in the hospital?"

"What's the cost?"

I scribbled down the answers and followed up with questions on radiation. After I had all the information, I thanked her and hung up; this was rude, but I was in no mood for niceties. I did not even explain why I was seeking treatment in Hong Kong; again, Mary was too polite to ask or I cut her off before she had a chance to do so. I called Jane, another friend, asking more or less the same questions in more or less the same order; she had had surgery and chemotherapy. They had different doctors but went to the same hospital.

Unlike my father, both used private healthcare; those with the resources too anxious to wait for treatment in the public system would do that. The new Hong Kong government has encouraged citizens to buy health insurance to cut down its healthcare expenditure, young people go for it and

less so with those in my age group. The insurance companies charge high premiums for our age category and almost
always do not cover pre-existing illnesses; and many reject
us coverage outright. Some friends stay with the public system because it is inexpensive; others dig into their savings
to go to private healthcare if they cannot wait. Both Mary
and Jane paid about US $10,000 to take the tumor out when
it would cost them only US $30 if they had used the public
one. Ten thousand was not a small sum, but I was willing
to pay the amount to be with Father for the time he had left.

Last I called my cousin Theresa with the same opening
line followed by the same line of questioning; she straddled
the dual public/private system in her cancer treatment.
One has to wait a long time for any test in the public system;
Theresa had her tests and surgery done in a private hospital before she went to the government facility for radiation.
With the breast cancer biopsy report in hand, she received
immediate radiation treatment when the incision closed.
Radiation cost her less than US $150 when she would have
to pay thousands in a private clinic.

I felt more settled with the information in hand and was in
a mood to talk. Besides, Theresa is my cousin and we are close.
I told her the reason for going to Hong Kong for surgery –
to keep the scheduled visit to keep Father from knowing
about my breast cancer; she immediately exclaimed.

"You won't be able to keep it from him. Uncle will know;
you will have to be in hospital for a couple of days."

"I'll tell him I am taking a short trip to Macau." Macau, a
former Portuguese colony now part of China, is twenty-five
nautical miles away from Hong Kong.

"You'll be a basket case. You'll look awful after surgery. Anyone can see you're sick." This scenario coming from someone who had gone through the procedure had to be true. A child is always a child to the parent whatever the age; sixty-seven-year-old me was still the child-daughter to my ninety-four-year-old father. When I visited, he treated me like a kid urging me to eat more food at meals and reminding me to put on a jacket when I went out. It would pain him so much to know I had breast cancer, and to see me undergoing cancer treatment would be worse; it would be particularly hard on him at this end stage of his life not being able to help in his condition. Since he had cancer, he might even blame himself passing the genes on to me. The thought that he might not be able to take all these again surfaced. I did not want to be responsible for anything bad to happen to him. If there was no way to hide my cancer from him, there was no point going there. If I were not there, he would not have to see me in that condition; he did not have to know about the diagnosis.

I took a 180-degree turn. I picked up the phone and dialed Father's number. I was not known for diplomacy and went straight to the point.

"Pa, I am not coming back on Wednesday. Victor has something to do. We'll come for Christmas instead."

I was abrupt, yet the message sounded casual, like telling a friend I would not drop by in the afternoon. I did not know why I picked December for the time of the next visit. It was September; perhaps I estimated that treatment would be over by that time, or Christmas seemed a good time to visit family. I had to name a date anyway.

There had to be good reasons for postponing a seven-thousand-mile trip across the Pacific Ocean a few days before departure; the reason or excuse was ludicrous – "Victor has something to do." The message said nothing. It was sheer scapegoating. I had never mentioned Victor coming with me. If he were, he would have made the needed arrangements and not wait till the last minute to have to cancel the trip; this was not him.

When my father had a stroke almost twenty years ago, he lost the use of his left arm, and his left leg was much weakened; he had a live-in caregiver. His two sons were busy with work and family, and they alternated to take him out on weekends; otherwise, he remained mostly housebound. He looked forward to my coming because he had my undivided attention on these visits. We both loved the outdoors and had a terrific time wandering together in the parks, strolling on the beach, walking along the harbor front, circling the Victoria Peak summit, or taking a ferry to the neighboring islands. In the early years after the stroke, he was strong enough to hobble with the support of a cane on these excursions; in later years he needed the additional support of the helper's arm, and with his waning strength he needed a wheelchair. He enjoyed the outings, so did Winnie, the live-in caregiver. Pushing a grown man in a wheelchair was hard work but more interesting compared to looking after one in the house; sometimes she suggested places we could go.

Father was never the aggressive type; he was the best of patients, never acting out in ways I heard some did. This did not mean he was not smarting from the loss of independence. He told me more than once he had lost the prerogative to make decisions and had to go along with what others wanted him to do. On occasion I noticed the hired help ignoring him when he called for assistance and at times made him do things for her convenience, not his. Yet they generally got along quite well and for that I was grateful; she even treated him out for breakfast once in a while after he paid her salary!

Father was especially accommodating now that he had to depend on others for most of his needs. When I told him Victor had "something to do" I did not know what that something was and would not have had an answer if Father had asked; he did not. He knew Victor's "previous commitment" was not the reason for the sudden change of travel plan, it was something else; he told me as much when I got back. He also knew all too well there was no point pursuing the subject because I would not tell him any more than what I had offered, and if he had tried to get more out of me, I would not have cooperated.

That day Father did not confront me with further questions, nor did he attempt to change my mind. He wanted very much for me to be there; there were times he had even asked me to move back to live with him. He knew what I had decided to do was out of his control. If he could not do what he wanted to do, he would have a harder time getting another person to follow his wishes; he could not even get the hired help to always do what he wanted. Besides, he knew me better. I was strong willed; to convince me to do anything different after I made up my mind would be difficult if not futile, a waste of his time; I might even get upset and snap at him.

He acknowledged his acceptance in not so many words. "All right," he said.

He did not utter another word, but he did not hang up; I was at a loss for what to say, and I did not put the phone down either. One was as disappointed as the other with the change of travel plan, and there was nothing we could do about it. Each held on to the receiver knowing the other party was at the other end of the line and reluctant to let go. Silence followed. I did not know how long the silence across the ocean lasted; it was a long one. It could not go on forever; the exchange or lack of one had to end. Something had to be done, I had to do something.

"Good night, Pa. Sleep tight." I said in a quiet voice.

He did not answer.

The line went dead.

THREE

Getting Past Gatekeepers

The next morning, I called Dr. Gray's office to make the arrangements to treat my breast cancer; I also wanted to go over the biopsy report with the doctor and to learn more about the prognosis. I was anxious to get started on the treatment procedures as soon as possible and dialed his number at nine o'clock sharp the moment I thought the office would be open.

The automatic answering device is almost standard in every medical office; to be connected to the doctor's office only means activating the machine at the other end. The machine announces the doctor's name followed by a message along the following lines: "If this is an emergency and you need help right away, please hang up and call 911." Then it would give instructions on how to reach the person the caller wishes to speak with. "If you are calling for an appointment, please press one." "If you require a prescription, please press two." "If you need to speak to a nurse, please press three." But it never gives the number to reach the doctor! This setup saves on operating costs, screens the callers, directs them to the "right" person, and reduces hassles for the employees. Talking to a machine, however, is not exactly a pleasant experience, especially for a patient anxious to get help.

Following the instruction and pressing the number does not always guarantee getting to speak to the person one is looking for. More often than not, another recorded message kicks in telling the caller someone will be there to help momentarily; then silence at the other end or sometimes soothing hold music comes on. More and more, even holding the line is discouraged; the recording asks the caller to leave a message explaining the purpose of the call and the phone number, or it simply asks the caller to leave a number to be called back assuring the latter will keep his/her place in the queue. I am always annoyed when I get such a response.

This happened the morning I called Dr. Gray. I pressed one as instructed to make the appointment and a recording encouraged me to leave a number instead. I wanted to see the doctor as soon as possible and did not take the suggestion. There was no music from the other end of the line and the silence was regularly punctuated by a repeat of the earlier message to hang up. It became a tug of war between human patience and the automatic continuous do-loop of a machine repeating the message after a programmed interval. The human lost out to the machine; I gave up after half an hour and left my name, phone number, and the appointment request. I explained to the machine that I had canceled the trip to Hong Kong and would like to see the doctor to sort out local breast cancer treatment. Not long into treatment I learned that talking to a machine was standard practice in medical offices, and with practice I could speak "naturally" to the machine as if I was talking to a person.

I had hoped to see Dr. Gray to learn more about my cancer and treatment or perhaps to hear some comforting words. Seeking comforting words from this doctor might be a tall order. He was not unkind or unsympathetic, but he was not exactly the warm, fuzzy type. I was asking too much and was destined to be disappointed. Had I not been so abrupt or belligerent the day before, perhaps I might have gotten both the information and support from the doctor. I lost my chance and got none of the above. His gatekeeper did not give me the appointment to see the doctor; in fact, he disappeared into the shadows in the entire course of my cancer treatment.

When my call was not returned in the afternoon, I called Dr. Gray's number before his office was about to close. Again, I had to leave a message; this time the call was returned. Whoever it was at the other end told me, "Dr. Gray is not looking after you. You have to go to a specialist. He is not taking care of your cancer." This was not what I had expected. Medical specialization or compartmentalization seemed to have cut me off from the family doctor. I felt abandoned.

She added, she had been trying to arrange an appointment with the specialist and could not get through to the other party.

I understood that getting the appointment was one among her many duties and she had other responsibilities and other patients to look after; it might be some time before she could call the specialist again. It was never easy to get through to a doctor's office; if and when she did, the appointment time she got might clash with a commitment I had made earlier, though it was more than likely I would drop everything to go, whatever time or day it might be. I did not need the complication. More importantly, I was impatient to start treatment as soon as possible and did not want to wait. Besides, calling the specialist would give me something to do, a better alternative than sitting waiting for her to call back. I offered to help.

"I can do it. Just give me the number."

The caller readily obliged.

"XXX-XXX-XXXX, Dr. Brown." She enunciated the numbers slowly and spelled out the doctor's name. I wrote both down on the writing pad, repeated the name and number back to her to make sure I got them right, and put the pen down.

"XXX-XXX-XXXX, Dr. McEwan," she continued, a new number and a new name. I was taken aback but dutifully wrote the information down. She did not stop there; she gave me a third number and a third name, three numbers and three names in total. I did not know this then, but the numbers belonged to Dr. Brown, the surgeon, and the two oncologists or cancer specialists Dr. McEwan and Dr. Gold, not their real names. Dr. Brown would take the tumor out, Dr. McEwan would give me radiation, and Dr. Gold, chemotherapy or drug treatment.

Over the years I was rarely sick. If I had the occasional cold or flu, I let nature take its course and did not go to see a doctor. I followed the seven-days remedy, rested, and drank lots of liquid. I am not exactly a convert to naturopathy. I am a minimalist as far as seeking medical help and taking drugs are concerned. I saw the family doctor twice a year for physical checkups and had a blood test and mammogram taken annually, and I did not bother to ask for the results. I reasoned that the doctor would seek me out if something was wrong; no news on the test results was good news; silence meant everything was fine. What happened in the last few days proved that I was right. The distancing from medical intervention, however, did not do me any favor. I was clueless how the medical system worked and ill-prepared to navigate its territory when I needed to do it.

Readings on the web did suggest that cancer patients receive multiple kinds of treatments (surgery, radiation, chemotherapy) which would mean I would be seeing multiple doctors; I did not put the information together and expected to see one specialist. The nurse might have been speaking of these specialists in the plural all along and I failed to catch it. The expectation to see only one doctor might also have come from other readings on the web too. "Curing" cancer involves multiple treatments, with a patient using some procedures to the exclusion of others or receiving all the different treatments one after another in different successions. The specialists offering these procedures work together to decide on the best treatment approach and develop the best treatment plan for the patient; a team representative will explain it to the patient. If this is how it is done, I shall be talking to one doctor at least for the start, the front one. Some sites even mentioned that the patient and family members are involved in these deliberations. This was something beyond my imagination! When I came across this piece of information, I thought to myself how open and democratic! I do not know that involving laypersons in the exercise is an offshoot of the emphasis on patient-centeredness in contemporary medical practice.

The medical profession is held in high esteem, and doctors are very much respected. The doctors' superior medical knowledge and their ability to heal give the profession an aura, and in a society that increasingly values health they enjoy inordinately high social status, privileges, and control of the healthcare system. Eliot Freidson, in *Professional Dominance,* labeled this medical professional dominance. As societies become increasingly committed to equity, human dignity, and democracy, however, the medical profession and practice come under scrutiny and criticism. The critics point to some doctors' haughty attitude and behavior treating patients as inferior and dismissing their wishes and preferences. Perhaps to correct the situation, in 2001 the National Academy of Medicine in the United States singled out patient-centeredness as a touchstone in the delivery of good healthcare and ask healthcare providers to respect the clients. At the time I was not aware of these developments or the emphasis on patient-centeredness that prompted the inclusion of the patient and family in treatment discussions. In any case, I was never included in any such discussions.

Neither did I have the opportunity to enjoy the integrative approach with the doctors working together as a team to look after me. Cancer specialists working together is only the best practice implemented in cancer centers or in big hospitals, with these experts meeting regularly to discuss cases, not in small towns where medical practitioners manage independent offices, seldom and perhaps never talking to one another. My town is in the latter category; my three cancer doctors never met to discuss my case. Where a patient lives makes a big difference in how treatment is carried out. When I expressed my disappointment not getting this dream team at a cancer support group meeting, a member pulled me gently aside to console me, "There's no such thing in this town." The three names and numbers I got that day gave this away.

I noticed the lack of communication among the three doctors early on in the course of treatment; they were not always apprised of the treatment progress and did not have my latest treatment report. To protect myself I played the great communicator, faxing one doctor's report to the others. Doing this did not always guarantee the smooth flow of information; the purported recipients sometimes never got the documents I sent. Who was to blame? Doctors not doing their homework, or support staff inefficiency? I could not tell. A team approach might not completely eliminate this problem, but it could perhaps attenuate it.

Even after I finished the active cancer treatment phase, I continued to miss having a team of doctors working together, but for a different reason. I met with the three doctors individually once every three months after active treatment, and later once every six months and then once a year. Going to these medical appointments required energy, and effort, and more so for someone who had just gone through cancer treatment. I was not happy with the arrangement. I thought if I had such a team looking after me I would be dealing with the team spokesperson or representative rather than seeing three different experts, in three different locations, at three different times to check the same breast in the follow-ups. But I was wrong. I did not know until more than a year after the active treatment phase that a patient with a "dream team" of cancer experts still has to see each medical expert individually in the follow-ups.

To return to my story, I had a different problem at the time. Getting the three medical appointments was the priority. I called three medical offices, listened to the same questions ad nauseam, and provided the same personal information over and over and over again at not the best of times and in not the best of moods. Perhaps patients with a team of doctors looking after them would have an easier time; they would answer these questions only once. This was what I thought. I could be wrong, and I would never know.

"What's your name?"

Since my Chinese name is unfamiliar to Westerners, the question was inevitably followed by, "How do you spell it?"

Perhaps they did the same to someone with a Caucasian surname, again something I would never know.

"Date of birth?"

"Do you have insurance coverage?"

I often wondered what would happen if I had answered in the negative to the last question. Would the other party hang up on me or politely tell me the doctor could not provide me service? Since I had health insurance, the conversation continued.

"What's the insurance company?"

"What's the group number?"

"What's your ID number?"

I jumped this hurdle every time I called another medical office. A doctor friend once told me his private practice is a small business and he a small businessman. Academics are less crass; they are more diplomatic and label the arrangement solo practice. Whatever the term used, doctors with their own clinics have to have enough clients to make ends meet and, in my friend's words, have to watch their bottom line if not their profit margin. A doctor would not have told a patient this, nor would he be so candid if we were not such close friends. Doctors need the information on the patients' insurance and credit card numbers to make sure they will get paid for their services. I can understand. However, I could not wean myself from the idealistic image of the altruistic doctors portrayed in so many stories to find the line of questioning on my insurance and credit jarring.

I answered the same set of questions four times in trying to make the three appointments. One doctor, who would remain anonymous, had a two-stage vetting procedure for new patients. The person at the other end asked me the questions mentioned earlier, and when I asked for the appointment after the question-and-answer session, she answered, "This is the number to call: XXX-XXX-XXXX." I was surprised. I am not a paragon of patience, and at a time like this, this quality was especially in short supply. Almost immediately I thought, "Wasting my time!"

"With whom am I speaking?" I quietly asked, hiding my irritation.

She worked for the doctor but was located in a different office. I suspected she was with a telephone answering service screening new patients to see if they qualified for medical service. This doctor had two lines of defense with two sets of gatekeepers. When I called the office for the appointment, I answered the same set of questions all over again.

The medical frontline workers were polite but not particularly helpful or as warm as I would like them to be. The receptionist, and almost always a woman, announced the employer's name over the phone followed with a perfunctory "How can I help you?" I say perfunctory because I sensed no enthusiasm or feeling in their robotic voices. It sounded bored, something to be expected with a speaker fielding the same questions every day. When I asked for an appointment, she would ask if I was a new patient; since I was a new patient, she immediately flooded me with questions on my medical insurance. I did not like this pragmatic business approach. They were so different from the frontline workers in the other service sectors with the same responsibility to make sure that clients will pay; the latter usually come across courteous and welcoming, anxious to please, ready to accommodate, and eager to provide the services. I did not get this impression at the medical offices. Instead, I felt I was the suppliant begging for help and the employees were gatekeepers vetting my qualifications to see if I deserved the service. I might have been overly harsh on them in my misery at the time, but that was how I felt.

And there were rejections. Dr. Gray's nurse was not the only one to stop me from seeing the doctor; the medical oncologist's assistant denied me an appointment too. And similar rejections happened several times in the months to follow. It was hard for me not to get the help I so desperately needed, and there were times I felt their decisions to deny me service were arbitrary. For some unknown reason I could not understand, Dr. Gray's staff deemed me undeserving of his attention every time I asked to see the doctor. I could not and did not see the doctor during the entire treatment period. When the blockage was lifted with active cancer treatment over, the subject came up in a casual conversation with Dr. Gray's nurse while waiting for the doctor in the examination room; she said her colleague was wrong not to let me see the doctor. By that time, I knew it should not have happened too. Family doctors had stood by my friends going through cancer treatment, meeting with them regularly, going over the reports with them, and calling the specialists for clarification. How many cancer patients know the rules of the game or how to play them? I did not know what I was entitled to and just accepted what the medical employees told me. Had I known it was not standard practice, I would have insisted. I would not have been so alone or lost through it all. I would have had a doctor at my side.

Airlines, banks, businesses, and sometimes even government departments have asked me to stay on the line to evaluate the employee who provided help over the phone, but no medical offices have asked me to do that. Perhaps they should. I was so exasperated with one operator I spoke with that day, I believed she deserved to be reprimanded if not fired. She asked the usual set of questions.

"What's your last name?"

"Kwong," I answered.

"Spell it out."

"K-W-O-N-G," I said slowly.

"I can't understand you."

"K for king ... " I said it one more time with each letter followed by a word beginning with the same.

"What's your insurance?"

"KIPG."

"Say it again! I cannot hear you." She said it authoritatively, loud and clear. There was also a tinge of impatience if not irritation in her voice.

I said it again slowly, "K for king ... "

"Never heard of it. Look at your insurance card." She was shouting if not yelling at me over the phone.

I was reading from the insurance card and could not give her any different answer. I had provided the same information to all the other medical offices.

"That's the one," I insisted and repeated the name. Why did you not recognize it? Could it be your ignorance? I thought. I knew better even in my frustration not to say it aloud. After some back and forth, she accepted the answer and continued her interrogation.

"What's your insurance number?"

By that time, I had lost my cool and repeated the numbers slowly in a pitch matching hers.

"Why are you so rude?" she asked. I might as well have asked her the same question.

"I am not rude," I retorted, even though there was some truth in the accusation. I was reading the insurance card number a decibel or two above normal and the tone of my voice spoke a thousand words.

"Why did you shout at me?" she pursued. She asked the wrong question, giving me the opportunity to speak my mind.

"You had difficulty hearing me earlier. You could not make out what I was saying," I said coldly, on the attack.

She got the message; her tone changed and she stopped yelling. I cured her listening problem. She continued her questions in a more even tone, and when she finished she hung up before I could ask for her name.

A friend from London once remarked that I spoke the language with the "received pronunciation" on television. I do not know if I should take the comment as condescending or a compliment, but I have to agree with her. I learned English in a missionary school in the British colony of Hong Kong and picked up much of my oral skill listening to the news on the radio and watching news on television. I enunciate words slowly and clearly. Listeners generally have no problem understanding me over the phone, but some have difficulty when talking with me in person. They ask me to repeat what I just said; the rare ones even take it upon themselves to correct my pronunciation. I often wonder if they would do the same to a Texan, a New Yorker, or an Australian who speaks the language with a distinct accent. Probably not. More likely these self-appointed language instructors would comment on the speakers' accents behind their backs. Why did they take it upon themselves to correct my pronunciation? I wonder if my yellow skin, slanted eyes, and flat nose have something to do with it.

The phone connection was good that day, and the person at the other end of the line should have had no problem making out what I said. The personal information collected from the start, however, gave my background away to put her on the alert. A Kwong was unlikely a native English speaker, though in these days, with global migration and intermarriage, a Kwong could have blonde hair and blue eyes. Perhaps a barrier sprang up as soon as the listener learned my last name and her difficulty understanding me got us both frustrated. I never found out who she was. No one in that doctor's office has treated me in the same manner since.

I only talked with the receptionists over the phone on that day to set up the appointments; these initial close encounters with the medical system were not exactly smooth or satisfying. I had read too many stories of caring doctors overcoming difficulties, doing everything for their patients, to give me a rarified unrealistic picture of the profession, and worse still I projected the image onto everyone working in the system to set myself up for disappointment. I expected sympathy from the receptionists and felt let down when I did not get it from them. When they asked for insurance and other personal information, I resented the line of questioning when it was their job to do so. I was offended by the arrogance and impertinence of some forgetting that the medical office was no different from the world outside with diverse personalities, including the prejudiced. These limited experiences weaned me from my illusion of an ever-caring medical system and lowered my expectations from the healthcare providers. But it did not make me feel any less disappointed or less hurt.

I was ignorant of the workings of the medical system and unfamiliar with its rules. I did not know the rights of patients or what I was entitled to. I did not appreciate the latitude of the power of the frontline workers; they can deny or grant passage to doctors as they see fit. They are the gatekeepers in medical offices, which means they control a patient's access to medical care. I accepted these gatekeepers' ban on seeing Dr. Gray that day and in the days to follow, and I accepted similar turndowns from the gatekeepers in the other medical offices. I suffered the consequences of my ignorance and lost out on the services that should have been available to me and I should have gotten. If I were knowledgeable of my rights and privileges, I would not have taken their no for an answer. I would have been more assertive; I would negotiate and I would fight with these frontline workers. I would have gotten the medical help I wanted so much, and I would have had an easier time on this cancer journey.

FOUR

Outward Calm

I was surprised to receive the three phone numbers from Dr. Gray's nurse and wanted to know what these numbers were for, but I did not ask. This was typical of me. The reticence to ask questions stemmed from my training – parents telling me to be quiet and demure and schoolteachers telling me to shut up in class. They were giving the same message – do not speak up. My parents told me not to interrupt when the adults were talking let alone to take them to task with questions; this would be rude. Teachers expressed displeasure when students asked questions in class; this was almost disruptive behavior. Growing up posing questions to a superior was seen as inappropriate if not an untoward challenge to authority, the exact opposite of what children are told to do today – speak and stand up for yourself. I incorporated what I was told to behave accordingly. If I needed answers, I would not ask; I would look for information on my own.

What my parents and teachers said became part of me. I did not ask the nurse what the three numbers were for; neither did I ask if I had to call the numbers in any order. The first question crossed my mind when I was talking with her on the phone; the second came up later. When I hung up, I checked the doctors' specialties on the web and called all three the same day. I saw Dr. Shield, the surgeon, the following Wednesday and scheduled the operation to remove the tumor the Tuesday after; I saw Dr. McEwan, the radiation oncologist, the same week I first met the surgeon and she asked me to come back a month after the operation to receive radiation. Things seemed to be falling into place with the two procedures (surgery and radiation) that the family doctor suggested finally scheduled.

I did not get an appointment to see Dr. Gold, the medical oncologist. When I asked for a date to meet with the doctor, the person at the other end of the line did not answer. I could hear her tapping away on the keyboard.

"I cannot find your biopsy report." She said after a little while.

"Dr. Gray said he sent it," I replied. Rather, his nurse said she would pass it on.

"Did you have your surgery?"

"No," I answered.

"Come back after you have it done and bring the biopsy report."

She said it in an authoritative tone I heard so many times that day trying to book the appointments, but she came across with the most commanding presence of them all. I was cowered by her confidence and humbled by my ignorance. I hung up.

I thought I had the document in hand. I did not know there are many kinds of biopsy categorized according to the location of the tissue, the purpose of the biopsy, or the instrument used to extract the sample; hence the different kinds of pathology report. A breast cancer patient usually gets two pathology reports in the course of treatment – an initial one performed at the clinic and another one after surgery. The words "Pathology Report" were stamped on the front page of the document in hand; it was the initial clinical biopsy report with information on the tumor cells obtained by needle aspiration. The pathology biopsy report the receptionist was referring to comes out after surgery; it is a reliability check of the information in the first report and gives additional information on the margin (that is, the tissues around the tumor) and on the lymph nodes obtained during surgery. It can tell if the cancer has spread beyond the breast and identifies the stage of cancer; the oncologists or cancer specialists will use the information to develop the treatment plan (whether the patient should get radiation or chemotherapy or both).

Patients feel lost when they hear they have breast cancer and want to do something quick; I was no different. Dr. Gold's assistant might not be the most diplomatic or polite; she was following medical protocol when she asked me to wait after surgery was done to see the doctor when the information was more complete, then he would decide on the course of treatment. Any treatment plan or arrangement made prior to surgery is tentative and superfluous, subject to change. I did not know that and viewed her request for me to wait an affront holding me back on the road to recovery. I was peeved with her, and perhaps with the doctor too. At the very least I was disappointed.

Cancer patients want to start treatment as soon as possible; again, I was no exception. Readers may notice that the surgeon mentioned in this chapter is different from the one cited in the last one. I dropped Dr. Brown, the surgeon the family doctor initially recommended, because he could only see me in three weeks; if I had to wait three weeks for the first appointment, I could expect to wait a lot longer to have surgery. I would not and could not wait. I wanted treatment immediately. I asked Dr. Gray for another surgeon, and he referred me to Dr. Shield. This doctor agreed to see me right away, and I was more than relieved when he scheduled the operation the following Tuesday. I never looked at his qualifications or experience.

For the same reason I was grateful and happy when Dr. McEwan promised me radiation a month after surgery at our first meeting. Little did I know that scheduling radiation with the tumor still in me, the second biopsy not done, and the pathology report missing was a leap of faith. It could be like the blind men feeling the elephant to get a picture of the animal with the impressions of the animal way off. The pathology report might corroborate what's in the biopsy report, but there was a chance it might not. If it was the latter case, my action had real consequences. If the disease was more serious than what the initial biopsy report suggested, radiation would not be sufficient to kill the cancer cells; on the other hand, if the problem was less serious than what the initial report suggested, the treatment would be overkill and I would expose myself to unnecessary treatment with all the possible detrimental effects of radiation.

According to the accepted medical protocol for breast cancer treatment, I should have waited for surgery to be done and the pathology report out before committing to any treatment procedure; in my ignorance and impatience I did not. I was lucky that the pathology biopsy report confirmed the findings in the earlier one and I got the appropriate treatment. Dr. McEwan should have known the medical protocol and waited for the second biopsy report to come out before offering me the radiation. I did not know why she did it; perhaps, like Dr. Gray, she thought that radiation after surgery would be the appropriate treatment and was confident enough to set a date. If I was to fault her for her action, I was equally guilty. I was complicit and more than a willing partner in this arrangement. I left her office that day feeling good with the treatment arrangement in place.

News of getting cancer takes away a person's sense of normalcy; the individual feels lost, uncertain of what lies ahead. The diagnosis of breast cancer robbed me of my "normalcy," both tangible and psychological. It disrupted my daily routine. I dropped everything to deal with the problem when there was really little I could do. Scheduling the treatment appointments was perhaps my way to do something and an attempt to regain some sense of control in my life. The two scheduled appointments gave me some idea of what was to come in the weeks ahead. I felt more settled and perhaps even a little happy, if a person with cancer could be happy. There were also moments I was proud of myself to have made the treatment arrangements within such a short time, not knowing that I was making a mistake to commit myself to radiation at this time.

At the 9/11 Museum in New York, I listened to the recordings of the passengers on United Airline Flight 93 bidding their last farewells to those they loved moments before the plane crashed near Shanksville, Pennsylvania, in 2001. These innocent victims had to be very fearful witnessing what happened on the plane and anticipating what was to follow. My untrained ear, however, detected only a little tightness, not fear or anxiety, in their simple moving affirmations of love. My situation was not as dire as these passengers'. I looked composed, perhaps another legacy of my training, but I was really very anxious. Appearances can be misleading; vital signs do not lie. My blood pressure told a very different story from the seemingly unperturbed exterior. Nurses in both Dr. Shield's and Dr. McEwan's offices found my blood pressure sky-high – shooting thirty to forty points above my normal. I could not tell if I was riled up worrying about cancer, treatment, Father's condition, or all of the above. I did not feel anything different; I did not know I was worked up. But I had crossed the red line into hypertension. No wonder high blood pressure is considered a silent killer.

I did not recognize what was going on inside me. I was probably lost, anxious, fearful, weighed down with many negative emotions in the whirlpool of my subterranean consciousness well beyond my reach and without my knowing. I was ready and eager to do something, anything to rid myself of cancer, the sooner the better. In my desperation I preferred action, or at least the promise of action, to no action. I clutched onto any offer of help; changing surgeons and scheduling the medical appointments were expressions of the desperation. The latter did not reflect sangfroid or superior organizational ability as I might like to believe; it signaled panic and reckless haste.

Having the appointments in place did not get me out of the woods. I might feel calmer with what I had accomplished, but I was haunted by a different set of worries. I had had benign breast tumors taken out before; this time the tumor was malignant and the operation was for real. More than likely the surgical procedure would be somewhat different from the last two, and I was not as confident as I had been before. I feared the worst. Radiation was a complete unknown. I never had it; it was something new. What would it be like? Dr. McEwan told me I had to have twenty radiation sessions; this would take a long time. Would it hurt? Would it burn my skin? Would it give me fatigue? Would it give me blisters? These were the fallouts from radiation I had picked up on the web. The side effects of chemotherapy were worse, though. I had read so much about them and they did not sound good. I did not even want to think about them. Lucky for me chemotherapy was not in the works, at least not yet.

I would have surgery in a week; not a long wait, but the short wait was challenging just the same. The knowledge of something unwelcome in the future and not knowing when it will come is tortuous; it is going through hell. I had some idea of what surgery would involve and knew when it would take place, but waiting for something unpleasant and not exactly sure what will be involved is not easy either. It was purgatory, that is, going through the same tortuous suffering of hell with a date of deliverance. I was antsy and jittery, sitting on pins all week, and the week of waiting felt like years. I wished the operation was yesterday with the ordeal behind me.

In the interlude of waiting, I asked other questions. My friend Jane had chemotherapy after surgery; Mary and my cousin Theresa received surgery and radiation for cancer treatment; another friend, Agnes, went through both radiation and chemotherapy after taking the tumor out for her stage 1 breast cancer. I was to have surgery and radiation; at least, this was the treatment schedule for now. How did they end up with their treatment procedures? How did I come up with mine? My impetuous declaration to leave for Hong Kong had left me without expert guidance; it seemed I had blundered into my present arrangement. I did not know I had violated treatment protocol; even then I could not help wondering how the decisions were made in their cases and how mine were made.

Articles on the internet told me the doctors discussed among themselves to find the best treatment for the patient; had the three doctors talked about my case? Did they discuss and conclude that radiation after surgery was the best route? It was obvious they did not. Dr. Shield and Dr. McEwan offered me surgery and radiation on the spot; they had not talked with each other. Dr. Gold was not even on board; he was unlikely to be a participant if such a discussion had taken place between the other two doctors. Was my case so straightforward and clear that no discussion was required? I hoped so. And I could not help wondering what would have happened had I met Dr. Gold before meeting with Dr. McEwan. In the stepwise approach I adopted in scheduling treatment appointments, the first doctor I met provided treatment. Dr. Gold was the specialist in chemotherapy; would I be receiving chemotherapy after surgery had I met him first? I would never know the answers to all these questions. The lack of answers filled me with doubts; the uncertainties and possibilities tortured me.

Otherwise, everything seemed normal at home. I knew I had breast cancer and I did not feel any pain or discomfort; my suffering was more emotional and psychological.

Since I did not feel anything different physically, there was no reason to play sick and stop doing what I normally did. Besides, puttering around the house would take my mind off my cancer and worries; I continued to be the homemaker cooking, washing, cleaning, and keeping the daily routine of domestic responsibilities. Victor looked after the outside of the house; he cut the grass, watered the plants, trimmed the bushes, swept the driveway, and went about his usual business in the yard. When he was inside the house he sat in front of the computer or played on his smartphone. Victor and I kept to our routine as if nothing unusual had happened.

Keeping the daily routine was a front and normalcy was a sham. We never mentioned cancer in our daily exchanges let alone discussed the treatment options or what might lie ahead, but I knew cancer and treatment were very much on our minds; I know it was on mine. Something had changed. We no longer chatted as much or talked in the same way as before. Our communication was limited to the mundane essentials of everyday living. When anything was said, it was in hushed tones.

"We are out of milk; we should get some."

"Are you coming back for dinner? What time?"

"I am doing the laundry. Do you have anything that needs washing?"

Even in our usual down time after supper, nestling against each other in front of the television, we said very little. We stopped gossiping about friends or commenting on local scandals. We no longer discussed national news or argued about world politics. Gone were the bantering, joking, and verbal one-upmanship we pulled on each other. Gone were the scandalous tussles and horseplay unbecoming to our ages but which we were capable of doing when no one was around. We were subdued. We hardly smiled when our eyes met.

Since that day in Dr. Gray's office when I got the news of breast cancer, I had become the automaton programmed to fight it. I had no sadness, no yearning, no longing, and no wants. I was not aware of the subterranean undercurrents of emotions whirling inside; any feelings I had were bottled up deep inside me beyond my consciousness. But cancer or its treatment had taken over my daily life. I marked my days no longer by the dates on the calendar, but by medical appointments. I met one doctor, and then another; there was the day for the blood test, the day for the CT (computerized tomography) scan, and so on and so forth – prescriptions from the medical profession to get as much information as possible to prepare and facilitate the breast cancer treatment to come.

I could not remember the errand I was running that day. On one of these never-ending medical errands alone in the car, the lid on my pent-up emotion blew off and I do not know what triggered it.

I backed the car out of the garage and drove along the familiar streets of our retirement community. It was customary for drivers in the car to wave to neighbors walking along the street; I stopped doing that since the diagnosis. The houses rolling past were just backdrops of the passageway I happened to be passing through, and the occasional pedestrians on the sidewalk were faceless figures I did not recognize or care to acknowledge. The car windows were rolled up and the radio was not on; I could hear the monotonous refrain of the engine and the soporific rumbling of the tires rubbing against the asphalt, a fitting audio backdrop to my benumbed state of mind.

Suddenly the floodgates of emotions flew open. I do not know why. Perhaps too many emotions were stored inside and blasted the cap. Outward equanimity gave way to an uncontrollable crying hysteria. Tears gushed from the corners of my eyes and tumbled down my cheeks. I brushed the rivulets with the back of one hand while the other was on the wheel, only to splatter the briny liquid all over my face and some into my mouth. The deluge continued; my nose dilated, my lips quivered, and my chest heaved. I muttered, "Why did this happen? Why did it happen to me?"

Psychology books say sometimes patients are angry when diagnosed with a deadly disease. They feel it's not fair for them to get it because they have done nothing to deserve it. I never thought of it that way. I did not feel injustice or resentment with what happened. I accepted my breast cancer as one of those things that could happen in life and a challenge I had to deal with, as my parents had told me so long ago.

No one can pinpoint the cause of cancer. Some blame it on the cigarettes we smoked, the alcohol we drank, the asbestos seeping through the walls, or the pollutants in the air. I have never smoked; cigarette smoke irritates my throat and makes me cough. I do not drink; alcohol gives me a rash and itchy skin that keeps me up all night. I have never been near any disaster zones; I have only breathed regular air – something everyone does. Others say the cancer is in the genes. Father has cancer, I have it too, but my two siblings sharing the same two parents are all right. It's all a matter of chance. The medical scientists speak in terms of associations and probabilities; they cannot tell who will get cancer and who will not. I would not spend time figuring out something that experts cannot explain or find an answer to. I attributed my cancer to luck of the draw or fate. When I asked "Why me?" I was not seeking an answer. I was not talking logic. I was not crying for justice. My tears were not tears of wrath or resentment; they were the outpourings of the weak. The two words "why me" were not a question; I was wallowing in self-pity.

All this time I was hungering for solace and support, though I did not show it. I wanted someone to comfort me, but I put up a strong front and covered my vulnerability. I did not want Victor to know how bad I felt. It was hard enough for him to see me with cancer; to see me breaking down would upset him more and he would worry how I would hold up. I tried to convince him I was strong enough to take whatever came my way. If Victor were in the car, perhaps I would have held back my tears; since I was alone, I let go. All defenses or pretenses were down. I cried.

I wailed like a child and called for Father, "Pa, Pa." I worried about him and missed him. The thought that it might be too late to see him was always with me. That was not the only reason I called out to him. I became the child clamoring for a father's attention and turned to him – the only other person besides Victor whom I could trust and know would protect me. He might not be able to help, not from where he was and not in his condition; I did not even want him to know my problem. But it felt good to know there was another person I could count on. Like the hype of virtual reality where one enjoys sights and experiences one otherwise cannot reach, I took comfort turning to him even when he was not there or could not help if he were, and I reached out to him. I regressed to the little girl calling on her father for comfort and protection. For a sixty-year-old woman to do that was pathetic. I do not know how long I cried and drove.

Father was going through the last stage of cancer and perhaps the last days of his life. Thoughts of how he faced his challenges suddenly flashed through my mind. The threat of dying was always there; why would it not be the case when the doctor told him he had only two years to live? I had caught him, eyes fixed on the television, deep in thought, not following what was on the screen. Having the hard polyurethane catheter stuck in his penis, the softest part of a man's body, for six years was no fun. It hurt when he walked and when sitting in the wheelchair; it hurt more when this foreign object brought infection to his urethra and bladder. After some time, the tube cut into the organ to turn it into hanging flesh. Then there was the growing amorphous pain from the metastasizing cancer. He could not identify where it came from, but it hurt inside. He told me many times, "I do not feel good; you don't know." An understatement, and I knew. He said, "I try not to think of it," and often he didn't. He was always happy whenever and wherever his sons, his daughters-in-law, or his grandchildren invited him out. When his family could not be with him, he kept busy going out with Winnie, the live-in helper, to the park, to the restaurant, or to the grocery stores. He was an avid reader, but his eyesight had failed him. He was an excellent calligrapher, but his hands shook too much. He was a tennis player, but his legs would not cooperate. He turned to watching replays of old movies on the video recorder during the day, prime-time shows on television in the evening, and followed every competition in every sport. His enthusiasm was contagious. He got Winnie hooked on tennis and soccer matches and, like him, to root for Djokovic, not Federer, and Manchester United, not Barcelona. He was always smiling when he ran into my friends on the street, and they often remarked on how alert, upbeat, and strong he was in his nineties. Images of him belted in a wheelchair, smiling and enjoying whatever he was doing, paraded in front of my mind's eye. My mood switched abruptly as I saw these pictures in my mind. If my ninety-year-old father with terminal cancer could take it so well, how could I feel bad for myself? I had no pain or discomfort. The clinical biopsy report had not identified the stage of cancer, but Dr. Gray's proposed treatment procedures coincided with those prescribed for a stage 1 or 2 of the disease. I felt ashamed of my self-pity. I told myself, "I am his daughter; I can do it. I will take cancer in my stride."

This might have been the first time my defenses caved in, but it was not the last. Time and time again on this cancer journey I was overwhelmed with self-pity and more and more with frustration at what had happened, anxious with what was happening, and fearful of what would happen. If Victor was around when these feelings came up to take over me, I would steel myself and remained calm; appearing calm really meant being withdrawn, morose, grouchy, and at times even cranky. If I was alone, I wallowed in self-pity and cried. Each time the thought of Father fighting his more difficult battle would spring to mind, each time I made a resolution to emulate him and to be equally brave in my own struggle with breast cancer.

FIVE

Excision

Dr. Shield, the surgeon, looked debonair in the photograph on his website. He had on a light blue shirt, a red tie, and a dark jacket matching perfectly with his dark hair and big, dark eyes. He looked approachable with a big smile on his lips; I felt comfortable having someone like him looking after me. Some doctors do not put their picture on their website; perhaps they are not as handsome or attractive as this one. Nonetheless, they almost always provide information on education, specialties, work experience, and sometimes patient reviews. When the last is available, the reviews are unfailingly positive. A few doctors give only the contact numbers, addresses, office hours, and the insurances accepted without any personal details; when personal information is not provided, it can be easily found on websites like Healthgrades, WebMD, and others.

In my impatience to obtain treatment I picked Dr. Shield because he was the first one available to see me. I was more than happy to find he had impeccable credentials. He graduated from a top medical school in the Northeast, spent some years at the prestigious Johns Hopkins Hospital, and had fifteen years of work experience. I would not trust my body to someone fresh out of residency or to an elderly surgeon with shaky hands. Dr. Shield had good patient reviews; they found him responsive to queries, helpful, and compassionate. One patient thanked him for resolving her GI problem when other surgeons had failed her. If he did so well in a delicate GI operation, he would have no problem removing a tumor from the breast. It never occurred to me that surgery on different parts of the body requires different skills and there is a specialty called surgical oncology. He was in general surgery.

Surgeons split their time between operating in the hospital and seeing patients in the office; consequently, the two workplaces are often in close proximity. Dr. Shield's office was on the second floor of a medical building adjacent to Grace Hospital, where he had operation privileges. When the surgeon walked into the examination room with the nurse close behind him, I was in for a surprise. He did not have his spiffy shirt-tie-jacket outfit; he was in scrubs, light blue shapeless unisex top and pants, standard for medical personnel in the operating room, something he had on for every subsequent meeting. His skin shone with a tan, suggesting he had just returned from a holiday in the sun, which could explain why I got the appointment on such short notice; he probably held off appointments until he came back from his trip and I caught him at the right time.

His persona was quite different from my projection based on his photograph. I had expected to meet someone sociable and outgoing; he was far from that. He turned out to be a man of few words, serious, quiet, and reserved, and I would even label him shy. He was very cautious. Michelle, his nurse, was a fixture at his side in every meeting and, my guess, a precaution taken examining a female patient who would bare her breasts every time. He was not the man of my imagination, but good looks and sociability are tangential to the quality of the medical care to be delivered.

The doctor gave a brief introduction on breast cancer and treatment, something the other two specialists also did at their first meetings, each emphasizing the procedures they were to be involved in. Dr. Shield's presentation was not interesting or engaging; I would rank his the lowest among the three. He repeated information I had learned from the web and assured me that I would come out all right, again something I already knew or believed based on my reading and Dr. Gray's proposed treatment plan.

His next question caught me by surprise.

"Do you want a lumpectomy or mastectomy?"

This was the first time a doctor asked me to pick a treatment option. I did not know about patient-centeredness; he was practicing it by consulting the patient. I was 100 per cent behind this democratic attitude, but he had overestimated me; I did not know enough about these procedures to take advantage of what he offered. Perhaps he should have explained the difference between the two.

My impulsive, foolhardy behavior to stick to the sched-uled Hong Kong visit had cut me off from Dr. Gray; no one had explained to me anything about cancer or its treatment let alone the alternatives. I had come across the two terms on the web and knew that the tumor is taken out in a lumpec-tomy and the whole breast is removed in a mastectomy. The choice between the two procedures rests on the size of the tumor and how far the malignant cells have spread – if the tumor is small and the cancer cells localized, one chooses lumpectomy; if it is large and the cancer cells in the tumor have spread widely within the breast, mastec-tomy is the better choice. What I knew came from the web, and I had begun calling these websites my web doctors, but the knowledge was generic. I did not know the size of my tumor, though I presumed it was small; nor did I know if the cancer cells had spread. I presumed they had not. There was really no basis for me to make the choice.

The web doctors mentioned another consideration in picking between the two alternatives: history of breast cancer in the family. A family history of breast cancer sug-gests that the patient may carry the gene to make him or her susceptible to the disease. I say him or her because men can have breast cancer too, though their chances of get-ting it are low compared to women. If the person carries the gene, he or she may opt for a mastectomy even with early-stage breast cancer. The celebrity Angelina Jolie car-ries the BRCA1 gene, which increases her probability of getting breast cancer, so she had a double mastectomy to remove both breasts when she was not even diagnosed with the disease. I found her preventive action drastic. It was not that I cared about looks; if I did, I could always have breast reconstruction like Angelina Jolie and ended up with better-looking breasts than my own. Since I had not known anyone in my family to have had breast cancer, it was not likely I carried the gene.

I am conservative when it comes to medical intervention. Leave well alone is my motto; the less intrusive the procedure, the better. Getting a mastectomy did not seem to offer any special advantage over the more conservative approach of a lumpectomy, so my choice seemed clear.

Dr. Shield was waiting for an answer. I thought I had come to the right conclusion and picked the less radical approach.

"Lumpectomy," I said.

I should have asked the surgeon to explain the two procedures, the pros and cons, and to give me advice; it never occurred to me to do that. It was my habit to answer questions I was asked, not to pose my own, in such situations. This did not help me to make the right decision.

I thought a lumpectomy was less intrusive and less radical, and to be fair it is. But I did not know that I would not need radiation if I had a mastectomy; I learned this only when the treatment was over. The surgeon might have told me, though, had I asked him to elaborate. Had I known that I could avoid radiation with a mastectomy, I would have seriously considered this alternative. I had already made one mistake on this cancer journey when I unwittingly violated medical protocol by scheduling radiation before I had surgery; now I made another – I made a decision with incomplete information. With the complications from radiation and the ordeal to follow, something I describe in later chapters, I lived to regret the decision.

If the surgeon had a preference for one or the other procedure, he did not show it. He went straight into the details of doing a lumpectomy. "We'll do that. I'll go into the sentinel lymph node to make sure that the cancer isn't there," he said.

A sentinel is a guard, the first line of defense, and the sentinel node is the lymph node closest to the breast; a person has more than twenty such nodes in the armpit to filter the lymph fluid from the breast. During the operation the surgeon takes out the tumor, the band of tissues around it, and the lymph nodes until the latest one taken out is clear of cancer. A cancer-free node suggests that no malignant cell has escaped beyond this point. Surgery is both remedial and diagnostic. It removes the cancer and checks its spread; that's why a breast cancer treatment plan (whether a patient should receive radiation or/and chemotherapy) is made only after this step.

"I'll close the incision with a plastic surgery technique," Dr. Shield added, almost as an afterthought.

I had come across "lymph node biopsy" on the internet but nothing on how a doctor would close an incision. Surgeons usually sew the opening with threads made from various materials; plastic surgeons close it with glue to leave little to no scar. Like much of my knowledge on cancer and treatment, I learned about these differences after the fact.

Dr. Shield was telling me what he would do to close the incision, not asking for my preference; his proposal sounded attractive. Using a plastic surgery technique to close the incision would give me a good-looking breast after a mutilating surgical procedure, so why not? I seconded his suggestion with my silent consent.

At seven o'clock on Tuesday morning, Victor and I were at the reception desk of Grace Hospital. After completing the paperwork, we were ushered into the pre-operation room, a long, narrow room with a row of twelve cubicles on the right facing the pale blue wall on the left. Each cubicle was large enough to accommodate a bed with a head table on one side and a chair on the other, separated from the neighbors on each side by a sky-blue cloth partition, and a drape of the same color at the entrance provided another modicum of privacy. Three cubicles were taken, and I had the one across the nursing station.

A plump woman with a round, ruddy face topped by a crown of curly brown hair walked into my cubicle. Her light green scrubs told me she was not a doctor; more than likely she was a nurse. She gave me a big smile and looked so pleasant I immediately took a liking to her.

"How are you doing today, sweetie pie?" She inquired.

As soon as the last two words left her lips I cringed. No one had called me that, not Victor, not my parents, not anyone close to me, and certainly not someone I met for the first time! Neither had I used it on anyone before, or since. If I were to use it, I would save it for cute little children, not a sixty-plus woman. I was taken aback, though I did not like her any less; I knew she was trying to cheer me up and put me at ease.

Over the course of cancer treatment, I was inundated with "darling," "honey," "sweetie," "sweetheart," and a host of other such terms of endearment from healthcare providers I had never met before and was not likely to meet again. As time went by, I got used to these forms of address and stopped reacting when someone gave me a sugary greeting. These attempts to calm patients might have worked with someone brought up in North America, not with me raised in the reserved Chinese culture. I wondered if this approach would work on a German, a Finn, or a person coming from a less emotionally effusive or less expressive culture. And how would they address men? Would they call them "sweetie pie" too? I was curious to know, and to know how those recipients would react.

If an unfamiliar casual address can make me feel uncomfortable, I can appreciate the variations in patient reactions to how they are received in medical offices and how important it is for doctors to know their patients. Kleinman may be speaking about psychiatrists when he says doctors should know and understand their patients to find the best cure, but it is true for all specialties. I think medical associations ask doctors to take patients' preferences into consideration in treatment decisions for the same reason. And it may be for the same reason too why some patients seek out doctors of the same ethnicity because these doctors generally understand them better and they feel more comfortable.

"What is your name?"

"What's your date of birth?"

The friendly nurse continued with questions that I soon learned to expect in these situations. She was making sure she had the right patient. She did not stop there. She asked me for the treatment procedure I was coming in for to make sure the hospital would not take out a wrong organ, the wrong breast, or do something not meant for me.

After these precautionary questions, the nurse left the cubicle for me to change into the patient gown with the opening in the front and returned to check my vital signs. My blood pressure spiked sharply, way above the normal 120/80 count, again betraying the stress deep beneath my composed surface. She secured a needle a little above the wrist on my outstretched right hand and connected it to the intravenous drip hung from a pole at the corner of the bed.

Victor sat mute in the chair beside the bed, and I amused myself by eavesdropping on the conversations in the next cubicle. A man and two women were talking about a party over the weekend, the savory steak the host offered, the fine wine Lorne brought, and Johnny's funny jokes. They were a jolly group and seemed not too worried about the procedure whomever was coming in for.

The next compartment went quiet. Victor left to run some errands, and I passed the time by peering through the gap in the front drape and watching the nurses at work – answering phone calls, filling out forms, filing papers, coming and going for I did not know what.

A young woman wearing rose-colored lipstick but otherwise with no makeup pulled aside the drape to join me in the cubicle. She was soft-spoken and introduced herself as Dr. Chris Jansen, the anesthetist. She wanted to know the medications I had been taking, if I had any allergies, and lastly, if I had any question for her. Doctors had asked me the last question before and each time I could not think of anything to say; I felt stupid. At the time I had not read neurosurgeon Henry Marsh's memoir *Do No Harm* and did not know that the query is pro forma not to be taken literally; it is a signal for patients to leave. I felt a little better after reading this when I could not think of any questions to ask. Dr. Jansen was the exception. She seemed to mean it, and she was persistent. When I did not have questions for her, she tried another tactic to solicit information. She asked me if there was anything else she should know. I did not know what she was after. I was not in a good mood on a day when I was to be cut up, and lying on the bed in the cubicle for hours did not help. Her question irritated me. Strange question! I thought. I could have said "stupid question." How would I know what she had to know? I only knew she would put me to sleep during the operation. If I knew what she had to know, I would be the doctor. I would not be on the bed. I was not being fair. She was cautious, doing her job, asking questions a doctor would ask anyone in this situation, but I was in a sour mood and did not appreciate her repeated attempt to solicit a response.

After another long wait, a friendly young man with a jovial face in a doctor's blue scrubs walked into the cubicle. He was bubblier and more talkative than the anesthetist. He gave me his name, which I forgot the moment he told me. He also introduced himself as the doctor to prepare me for the operation. What would he do? He did not explain; neither did I ask. Again, I learned afterwards from the web that this "preparatory doctor" was the diagnostic radiologist to locate the tumor the surgeon was to take out. He did not ask if I had any questions for him, which I appreciated. I was spared from the meaningless if not futile exercise that only exposed my ignorance and irritated me. If he did ask, he would get the same answer. I had none.

My bed became a gurney with the intravenous bag hung on a pole anchored to the bed and the "preparatory doctor" pushing it. I was surprised to see this young man doing the transfer. This would have never happened in Hong Kong with its very strict hierarchical social protocol shaped by the conservative British and Chinese cultures; only an orderly or someone in the lower ranks would do the menial task. The young doctor did not seem to mind it one bit; on the contrary, he seemed to relish every moment of the exercise. He pushed the gurney with great gusto, skating and skidding along one narrow corridor after another, one quick sharp turn to the left, another to the right, rounding more corners and racing down more narrow pathways. I felt dizzy and nauseated, with the ceiling receding fast overhead and more so with each sharp turn. I closed my eyes. My left hand gripped a pole of the bed guard; the fingers of my upturned right hand with the IV stuck in it squeezed the bed sheet underneath. Luckily the nurse taped the cannula securely and it withstood the rough ride. And lucky for me too, no one came in the opposite direction when we were racing in the warren of narrow passageways. I could not imagine what would happen if someone did; there would be a head-on collision and I, the casualty.

I was not dazzled to have a doctor pushing my hospital bed; instead, I was sickened physically by his reckless run on the track. I heaved a big sigh of relief when we came to the finish line, a small room with an imposing machine standing tall, almost touching the ceiling. I did not know what the equipment was for; we never used it. I only felt crammed as if I was in a closet with this gargantuan against the wall hovering over me in such a small space. The young man whose name I forgot seemed to have enjoyed himself thoroughly; his cheeks were flushed and his eyes shone.

The diagnostic radiologist gave me a shot. He did not tell me what he had injected in me; it could have been radioactive blue dye to locate the lymph node to be taken out or something else. He left the room for the drug to go where it's supposed to or to take effect, and he came back to tell me I would feel a little discomfort with what he was about to do. The procedure gave more than a little discomfort. I could not see what he did while I was lying on the gurney. I felt a prick on my right breast; most likely he punctured the skin to thread something in. The thing wriggled inside my breast, causing me pain each time it moved, and I flinched and tightened my muscles waiting for the next move. He was performing wire localization – sliding a wire with a hook at one end to grab the tumor in the breast. The wire was encased in a narrow hollow casing to be removed after the hook was secured. When he thought he had anchored the hook and pulled, what should have stayed came out.

"I am sorry. I have to do it again," he apologized.

Common courtesy would have me say some polite words like "It's OK" or "Mistakes sometimes happen." I would have done it under different circumstances. But I was not in the mood to do so. I would not make him feel better for what he did to me; he would be doing it again and I would feel pain again. I bit my lip and kept my silence.

He repeated what he did and got the wire secured. Mission accomplished.

"These doctors look so young; I wonder if they know their stuff."

My uncle made this comment when he was in the hospital. It sounded funny to hear him say that at the time. Reverse ageism! Fixation on the long-held Chinese cultural belief that the old necessarily know everything and are always right, and the young can never match their knowledge or wisdom! I laughed then. Now it was my turn to wonder if this young doctor-athlete who raced down the track knew his stuff, and the idea of young doctors not fully prepared didn't appear so funny now that I was on the receiving end. The doctor looked barely thirty; he probably had the book knowledge but not the hands-on experience of his more seasoned colleagues. I might be among his first guinea pig patients to hone his skill.

The preparatory doctor pushed me through another labyrinth of narrow corridors, this time at a much slower pace. The mistake he made in the closet room probably sobered him, and I had a smoother ride to the operating room. The anesthetist was perched on a table in the corridor looking completely relaxed, head bent and legs dangling over the edge; one palm was tucked snuggly between her behind and the table, and the other supporting a smartphone with her thumb deftly swiping its surface. My immediate thought was, "How unprofessional!" I stopped myself. She was not on duty in the operating theater. We belonged to different generations. The anesthetist, like the diagnostic radiologist, looked barely thirty, and I was double her age. She probably used her phone to do banking, to shop, to get in touch with friends, to play games, to watch movies, to buy coffee, and to perform a host of other activities. I used mine strictly as a phone.

The operating room was nothing like the spacious operating theaters seen on TV with the operating table in the middle; one or more big overhead surgical lights above; impressive machines with wires, dials, and monitors sitting on the side; cabinets full of equipment against the wall; surgical instruments neatly arrayed on trays; and the nurses standing by ready for action at a word from the doctors. My operating room was in keeping with the back corridors and back rooms I had been in all day – small, with the gurney taking up almost a third of the space and a few consoles and trolleys resting haphazardly along the wall. With no operating table in sight, I presumed the gurney would serve as the operating table as well.

A nurse in gray scrubs was hovering over a tray of surgical instruments when Dr. Shield walked in; it was the only time I did not see Michelle, his nurse, at his side. He did not greet me or acknowledge my presence; I had become the body on the operating table to work on. The anesthetist followed closely behind with her phone nowhere in sight. Five steps past the entrance, she was at my side. She asked me to extend my left arm and poked a needle in it; I was out in seconds, missing the most important part of my day's activities.

When I came to, I was resting on the bed in the pre-op room, now my post-op room, or was it the same recovery room where the nurse monitored my vital signs when I was unconscious after surgery? I would never know; it did not matter. Victor told me Dr. Shield had come out two hours earlier to tell him the operation went well. I did not know where I was in that intervening period.

The same pleasant, plump nurse with the sweet face who helped me in the morning came to tell me I could leave. I nudged my elbows against the mattress to slowly push the torso up and reached the railing for support to move to the top of the bed; I stopped when I could go no farther and rested against the headboard. The nurse noticed my lethargic movements and asked if I would like a drink of water. I nodded not because I needed it; in my grogginess I assented to any suggestion. She brought me water in a paper cup and I gulped it down. Before she could pull aside the drape to leave, I threw up. I had not taken anything since the night before; the vomit was clear. The nurse turned her head to take one look and came back with a small plastic basin. I sat on the bed with the basin on my lap until the retching subsided. It was past four o'clock in the afternoon when I waited outside the hospital entrance in a wheelchair with the plastic basin on my lap for the ride home.

When I saw Dr. Shield a week later in his office, he told me the tumor was out, the margin was clear, and the lymph node carried no cancer cells. That was good news. I was clear of cancer. I could have peace of mind. Every minute of the long nine hours spent in the hospital seemed worthwhile. The worst was over. Or so I thought.

SIX

Fatigue

After surgery I had pain at the incision and in my right shoulder; the former went away in a couple of weeks, but the latter stayed to keep me up at night for months. Dr. Shield gave me a prescription for hydrocodone to kill the pain when the effects of the anesthesia wore off. I bought the drug but never took it. News of the opioid epidemic was coming out, with patients taking painkillers and not stopping, getting hooked, and progressing to more potent addictive drugs; I did not want to take the risk of falling into the same trap to have to deal with an additional problem. I was resolute to tough it out, and my childhood training in stoicism helped.

In addition to the pain, I had no energy. I thought the physical and emotional stress of going into the hospital made me tired and the feeling would go away in a couple of days, or at most a week or two; it did not. In the past my muscles ached after strenuous exercising; the sensation would disappear after a good night's sleep, or at most a couple of days, and I would be myself again. This time it did not; the tiredness stayed. I always thought fatigue was another word for being tired. This is probably not the case. Fatigue refers to the lingering, overwhelming, consuming listlessness and lack of energy for seemingly no reason; I experienced it for the first time after surgery and understood the meaning of the word. There was no muscle soreness, only the amorphous and persistent absence of strength and energy that would not go away.

Since I felt like this after surgery, I thought the procedure had to be the culprit, although I could not understand why such a minor operation with an incision of no more than an inch could wreak such havoc. Victor blamed it on the side effects of generalized anesthesia, and he might have been right; the web doctors where I got the information on breast cancer did say this could sometimes happen after surgery.

My energy and strength slowly returned in the weeks to follow; I felt a bit better, but I was not my normal self. Jumping a bit ahead of my own story, when radiation started my energy went down again, and with the complications in the procedure I became more enervated. The fatigue lingered after the active treatment phase and for a long time to follow. My energy came back very, very, slowly, and it was more than a year before I could pull myself together to start writing these pages. And I never fully recovered; I still easily tire.

Medical science has made great progress in the understanding and treatment of breast cancer, but the discipline continues to speak in terms of probability, not with the certainty of physical laws. Medical practitioners cannot anticipate all the different reactions to treatment. Even when a treatment has proven to be generally effective, one patient may respond positively and the cancer goes into remission, but it may not work on another and the tumor may continue to grow. Even when the treatment is effective at one time, it may cease to work after a while and the cancer grows again. Drugs usually come with multiple side effects; doctors cannot understand why some patients taking a drug have side effects and others do not, nor do they know why one patient develops one side effect among a host of possible fallouts and another a different one using the same drug. Medical websites acknowledge these variations and anomalies. Human beings are alike and yet so different; with so many variables or factors at play at any one time, no one can tell ahead which recipient will get side effects and which will not, or who will get what. It is not the first time, nor will it be the last, for me to read the following statement or something similar on reputable medical websites or in the literature: The reason is not known. There are many questions for medical science to answer.

My lingering fatigue is a good example. Surgery and radiation sapped my energy. Some patients, like me, are hit with fatigue, while others are not. A friend who had a mastectomy, a much bigger operation than a lumpectomy, did not feel tired. After the breast was removed, she went about her everyday activities waiting for the incision to heal and breast reconstruction to begin. Two friends went through radiation treatment, and one never stopped work; the other stopped work initially only to go back to her job because she was bored. They had had enough energy to do what they did and I had none. When I told one of them about my fatigue during cancer treatment, she pooh-poohed my concern and remarked, "Breast cancer is nothing." She was speaking from her experience, not mine.

Speedy Gonzales became Slow Poke. Before surgery I was quick and could take two steps before I said the word "one"; after surgery I probably counted to ten before I finished moving my two legs to make one step. My legs felt as if they were carrying weights or they were the weights. My every move made me think of the little old women and men with bent backs walking the streets of Hong Kong where I grew up. Their L-shaped bodies with torsos almost parallel to the ground reminded me of moving Allen wrenches and I worried they might topple. My young mind could not understand why they walked with such studied steps; now it's my turn to go so slow and I knew the reason. My back might not be bent; I made the same ponderous movements because I did not have the energy to lift my limbs or get them to go faster.

I no longer had the strength to do the usual housework and did just enough to get by. I did whatever I had to do with the greatest effort and with the same slug-like movements, and more often than not I did not have the stamina to finish what I started. Both the web doctors and friends suggested drinking juice to boost immunity, and I followed their advice. I have always liked fruit drinks, making them had been easy. It was not the same after surgery. Preparing it took half a day and another half a day for me to recover. To bend down to get fruits and vegetables from the bottom of the fridge, take them out, stand up straight, and take the few steps to put them in the sink required great effort. The ingredients were too heavy to be carried in one go, and I had to do it in a few expeditions. Then I had to wash the fruits, drain them, get a knife, cut them, get the juicer, throw the fruit pieces into the juicer, put the plug into the socket, and start the machine. Every move was a challenge. Fruits, cutting board, containers, and plates weighed like nine-pound shot puts and the juicer, a ton. My wrist was weak, and I had difficulty cutting even fruit. My legs did not cooperate; standing to wash, peel, cut, and blend the ingredients was too much, and I needed a chair when sitting was not the best position to perform these tasks. After juicing, there was the cleanup. I did not trust Victor to come up with the concoction, but I had no energy left by the time I finished the preparation and he did the cleaning. Once cancer treatment started, poor Victor worked both inside and outside the house. He was not only the gardener, the driver, and the handyman; he was also the grocery shopper, dishwasher, housecleaner, and errand boy.

When cancer patients complained that their arms felt stapled to their sides, I knew the feeling. If mine was not completely glued to my body, it was attached to a strong, heavy spring anchored to my waist; raising my right arm to do anything was a major struggle fighting the tension of the invisible spring's steel loops. Moving it a little too fast or pulling it a little too hard sent a jab to my shoulder; for my arm to reach the shelf at eye level was difficult; forcing it to go a little farther sharpened the pain, and to raise it any higher was impossible.

I stood on my toes to make myself a little taller to avoid overextending my arm and lifted it slowly to retrieve or deliver anything on the shelves over the kitchen counter. A plate, a glass, or a bowl felt heavy. To relieve the load on my right arm, my left hand sometimes held my right elbow to support and guide it to where it was supposed to go. I could have relied on my left arm to do these tasks and become ambidextrous, my right arm would have felt better, but I knew if I did that the muscles would atrophy, the range of movement would become more restricted, and the problem would get worse. I might not be able to move it again. I would not be ambidextrous; I could become a woman with one paralyzed arm.

Fatigue did not necessarily translate into a good night's rest. There were many times when I would wake up in the middle of the night and could not go back to sleep. Thoughts of what was happening surfaced and circled in my mind. I could not understand why my body felt that way and wondered if and when I would be whole again. I felt sadness, and again self-pity. I cried. When that happened, I sneaked into the next room so as not to wake Victor, turned on the computer, and pounded my thoughts away on the keyboard. On re-reading what I put down at the time, I was surprised to find the entries were not on my misery or physical discomforts as I would have thought; they were instead memories of the good times spent with Father. Thinking these thoughts could have been my escape from reality; Freud would see it differently and interpret this as my subliminal desire to be with my parent.

Sometimes I read when I could not sleep. I had stopped reading books because I could not concentrate and finishing one would be difficult with the lack of energy. Even in my illness I could not escape the habitual compulsion to finish something once I started; not being able to accomplish that made me feel bad. In addition, books felt heavy in my hands, so I turned to magazines instead; they were lighter and the articles shorter. The subjects in the periodicals did not necessarily interest me; most of the time I did not know what I was reading and could not tell what I had read, but going through the motion of reading calmed me. I would fall back to sleep after a while.

I had great plans before surgery. I intended to give the house a thorough cleaning because I would be housebound; some friends thought the same and made the suggestion. It would be autumn, not spring cleaning. This turned out to be wishful thinking; I did not even do regular house cleaning. Dust gathered on the floor, dirt covered the counters, grease dried on the stove, and scum lined the bathtub. Victor performed the bare essentials to make our living conditions tolerable and livable. Friends had thought I would use the time to read, but as I mentioned earlier, I did not have the interest or wherewithal to do that. I did not even turn on the radio or television. I rested a lot, which meant I did nothing. If I was not lying on the bed, I sat in the armchair hardly moving and staring vacantly ahead, seemingly perfectly content. In the past I would have been so restless sitting doing nothing; now I was perfectly comfortable with inaction.

It was fall when I finished surgery. At this time of the year, the Chinese flame tree and the Arizona ash turn gold and red in the front yard; soon they drop their leaves to expose the beautiful lines of their bare branches silhouetted against the clear blue sky. The leaves on the orange and pomelo trees in the backyard stay green on the boughs; their nondescript fragrant little white flowers shrivel, the petals fall, leaving the tiny ovules in the receptacles hardly visible to the naked eye. The little green globules swell, turning orange on one tree and yellow on the other, beautiful against the vibrant foliage nurturing them. In years past I would be admiring the evolving colors on nature's palette; I was practical too and counted with excitement the fruits hanging from the branches, watering them, fertilizing them, nursing them, and waiting impatiently for the harvest. Nature most likely put on the same display that year, but I hardly directed my eyes beyond the window or noticed anything when I did. I could not remember if we harvested anything, and if we did Victor was the one to pick them.

With complications developing during radiation, treatment time doubled and I remained housebound till the following March. There is no real winter in the South comparable to those in the North; autumn turns almost immediately to spring. The temperature starts to rise in February and tiny buds break out from the bare branches. Thoughts turn to love even for the birds. I have never witnessed these feathery creatures in their mating games; they guard their privacy, and I can only hear them rustling among the bushes. However, they share with me their avian courtship songs. In the early hours of the morning, they make a ruckus outdoing each other in their pleasant, though in my opinion not too romantic, love songs. The warblers give their shrill trill, the wrens add a few additional notes to their repertoire, and the mockingbirds are the loudest of them all. I marvel at how their little throats can sing so loud and carry on the tune, if one can call it that, for so long. After a while I pick my favorite and listen eagerly to the matinee performance amidst the cacophony. That spring the birds did not go silent, though I did not hear them sing. It was not what the literary lexicon called "pathetic fallacy," with nature sharing my mood to go on hold; I was simply deaf to all that was going on around me.

With complications in radiation and my energy dropping with each additional session of treatment my world shrank to the confines of the four walls of the house; as fatigue intensified it diminished further to the two-feet radius of the recliner where I sat in my waking hours. I was wrapped in my cocoon of self-imposed sensory deprivation entombed in a world of noiseless nothingness oblivious to the change in seasons and everything outside. I did not notice anything. I did not hear anything. I did not have interest in anything. I did not think anything. I did not do anything. I was content to stare, to sit, and to sleep. An outside observer might label me depressed at this time, and it would be easy to dismiss my behavior as such; however, I do not believe this was the case. I might have felt tired, not done much, and had no interest in things around me, but I do not believe I met the American Psychiatric Association criteria for depression. Besides, I have always believed the depressed person feels down and loses interest in the things around them, resulting in lethargy, not the other way around. I was drained of my strength after surgery, and the physical fatigue had elevated, or perhaps for a better word "reduced," me to this state of physical, mental, or emotional suspended animation. True, I did not do much, but what could I do in that physical condition? True, I was not happy, but who would be happy at a time like this? True, I worried, but who would not worry in this situation? I had no negative thoughts; I had never thought of killing myself. On the contrary, I felt content to do nothing in my waking hours. Being blank is perhaps the best word to describe the state I was in. Only with active cancer treatment over, when I gradually regained some strength, did I realize the deep void I had been living in.

SEVEN

Culinary Advice, Friendly Support

I left Hong Kong in 1967 to attend a university across the Pacific and stayed, but I remained in contact with friends via letters, then by emails, and had the occasional gatherings with them when I visited my parents every few years. The majority of my friends finished school, worked, married, and started their families in Hong Kong; they left only after the 1984 Sino-British Joint Declaration when Britain agreed to return the colony to China in 1997. In the years following the Joint Declaration they left Hong Kong in droves and in haste. My circle of friends was scattered all over the world; some went to England, others to Australia and New Zealand, many went to Canada, and some to the United States. Accustomed to living in a city of over six million people, they picked the large cities for their new home; none settled in the small town of 300,000 I was living in.

I had been living in America for more than forty years and made many friends. People brought up in the West are usually more outgoing compared with those raised in the very Chinese society of Hong Kong; it was easy to make friends at my university, in the workplace, or in the neighborhood where we lived, and we made more friends through friends. The majority of our friends were locally born Caucasians; others, like me, were immigrants from Europe, Africa, or Asia; and a few have become closer to me than my childhood friends. When Victor and I traded the cold north for the warmer climate of the south on retirement we left our friends behind. It was hard to make new ones when we did not go to school or work. Our neighbors were our age or a bit older and kept very much to themselves; we remained quite isolated with no childhood friends or adulthood friends, if there is such a term, living in town.

Elizabeth Edwards, in *Saving Graces*, and other cancer patients wrote about the flowers they received, the casseroles neighbors brought, and the stream of visitors dropping in to wish them well when they were receiving cancer treatment. I got none of these. I was not envious. I am allergic to flowers; my friends knew that, and they would never bring me bouquets. If anyone did, I would give them away the moment the gift-bearer left the house. As for casseroles, my friends, like me, were not the homely type. Some would not know how to make it, and others would not bother; if they brought food, more than likely they brought restaurant takeout. With no friends living close by, none came knocking on our door; if anyone did, I would be too exhausted to enjoy the company. My neighbors might have brought me flowers, made me casseroles, or visited if they had known what was going on, but they did not know. They were advanced in years and I did not want to trouble them; I never told them my medical problem.

Solace came from the support group sponsored by the local cancer society. I attended the meetings every two weeks. All fifteen members in the group had different types of cancer, in different stages, or suffered it at one time or another. Two finished cancer treatment and they were still experiencing fallouts from the treatment procedures. One had muscle pain and numbness in the hands; the other suffered brain fog. The rest were coping with treatment and taking the challenges in stride. One member with stage 4 lung cancer would not give up signing up for one clinical trial after another that had kept her going for a few years. Another with metastasized stomach cancer held on to his job to feed his young family. Two women walked around with their hairless heads nonchalantly; one looked so chic in her fashionable hats and coiffure wigs. Their courage and optimism, especially among those in late-stage cancer, were simply awe-inspiring; no casual observer would recognize their challenges and know what they were going through. They were my role models and inspiration, and I recognized that my problem was nothing compared to theirs.

We knew each other's first names; otherwise, we knew little about each other except that we had cancer and whatever additional information came out in the course of our exchanges, which could sometimes be very personal and intimate. At our bi-weekly meetings, we talked about what we were going through, our physical discomforts, our feelings, and how we tried to cope. One member complained a lot; when she did that the rest of us quietly listened because we understood the need to vent. Another said time and time again that she did not have energy and would stop exercising, and every time she said that someone in the group would praise her efforts for walking with the walker in the garage and encouraged her to continue. When I lamented the absence of a dream team of specialists to look after my breast cancer, a comrade comforted me and gently informed me that this arrangement was not available in town.

There was a strong sense of camaraderie among us. We understood what the others were going through and cared for each other's well-being. We trusted each other and were candid at the meetings. We told our stories and said what we thought. We helped each other in ways we could; we shared information, elaborated on coping strategies, and gave suggestions to the problems anyone raised. We were never judgmental in what another did or thought; and if we disagreed, we would gently provide another view to be considered. Even this reserved Chinese woman felt comfortable enough to open up; I did not hold back to tell my problems, my fears, and my anxieties. I found the exchanges at these meetings so rewarding and useful that I never missed one. In fact, attending these meetings was my only social activity during the course of treatment.

Juanita, a member of the group, complained that her friends disappeared once they knew she had cancer and called them fair-weather friends; the others comforted her, telling her that sometimes people did not know what to say and stayed away for that reason, not because they did not care. I recounted my not-too-different reaction when my friend John told me he had throat cancer on the phone. I was taken by surprise, did not know what to say, and talked about something else. Juanita was not consoled by my story. I never told her I called John, who lived in a different city, regularly afterward to see how he was doing.

When I told friends of my breast cancer on the phone, their reactions were not too different from mine when I learned about John's throat cancer; they were taken aback and at a loss for words. One gave a response I would never have expected. She exclaimed, "Hoo! How did you get that?" with shock in her voice. I did not know how I got cancer and had no answer; I might have taken it to mean she was blaming me, though I knew she did not mean it that way. The responses of other friends were not so awkward; nevertheless, I could detect the discomfort groping for the "right" thing to say. Really, how many "sick" friends does a person have to have in order to know how to behave at a time like this?

I am a private person and told only close friends about my breast cancer, or it came out when someone specifically asked how my health was doing. Indeed, some friends who should have been informed did not know of my illness and expressed surprise when they heard of it much later after treatment was long over. However, once a few friends knew, friends told friends, and news of my cancer spread. My generation of friends might have embraced the technologies of the digital age to email or text each other and do FaceTime with their children and grandchildren; when it came to inquiring after sick friends, calling over the phone seemed to be the medium of choice.

Out-of-town calls kept coming in. It might be draining to take these calls, but talking on the phone was a welcome break from the monotony of being confined in the house. The callers were solicitous, wanting to know how I was doing. They were sympathetic and concerned and wished me well. Religious friends offered to pray for my speedy recovery; I did not belong to any church groups, but I appreciated their kind gestures just the same. In these phone conversations we talked about cancer as well as other subjects. I enjoyed the latter more than the former because it took my mind away from what was happening.

I confided my worries to friends. Sharing my concerns with those who had cancer was like talking to members of the cancer support group, kindred spirits who knew what I was going through. Telling my woes to friends who had never had cancer could be equally satisfying; they were understanding and expressed their empathy in not so many words. When I was unhappy with the radiation oncologist and debated switching doctors (something I will elaborate on later), Emily listened, acknowledged I had a problem and a tough decision to make, and warned me that I would probably second-guess whatever I chose to do. When I complained of the difficulties keeping house in my condition, Parvin reminded me that many women with breast cancer had young families.

"At least you don't have kids to look after. Think of the women with cancer and young children to care for!"

She was forthcoming. She reminded me there were many others in more difficult situations and told me to put my problem in perspective. She pulled me out of my self-absorption and set me straight. She was a true friend.

There were times I did not pick up the phone because I did not have the energy or the mood to chat. The reluctance to answer calls increased when I grew more tired with each radiation session, and when complications developed I became totally exhausted. The phone ringing woke me up from my nap. Without thinking, I fired off an open email telling friends to stop calling. It was rude to do that. A Caucasian friend mentioned later in passing that my email was "interesting"; she was being diplomatic. Chinese friends would have found the missive offensive; even in the brain fog of my illness I knew better than to send them a copy. I was right. A Chinese friend gasped when I mentioned what I did; another agreed with me that my Chinese friends might not have been able to take it. Perhaps even a few Caucasian friends were offended and never called again.

Most friends respected my wish and stopped calling. Before long, though, the phone started ringing again. My friends were worried. The caller almost always started by asking, "Are you in the mood to talk?" or something to that effect. It was an acknowledgment of the earlier do-not-call message I sent, but they cared enough about me to want to know how I was doing and to risk rejection. I was touched.

In a poor country with scarce resources, food is important. In the past, eating da yu da rou (big fish and big meat) was a symbol of wealth in China. Hosts offered their guests many dishes, with lots of food left untouched at the end of a meal to show their hospitality and to show off their wealth. Even after Hong Kong became a cosmopolitan city, food remained central to the social culture. Chinese love food. When friends get together, they have to have a meal, if not a banquet – the more courses the merrier, the more sumptuous the dishes the happier, and for the host, the more food left on the table after the meal, the prouder they feel. My Chinese compatriots with this wasteful habit do not make good stewards of planet earth.

Eating nutritious food is especially important for a person recovering from an illness. My Chinese friends offered me no shortage of advice on the subject. They warned me to stay away from beef during convalescence because it is "re," or hot. They were not talking about temperature but something more abstract like yin and yang; "re" has to do with the balance of heat and cold in the body, something I do not pretend to understand and shall not attempt to explain. I was not to eat anything "du," literally translated as poisonous, but it doesn't mean something that will kill me either; it simply means something that is not good for me. Duck and lamb fall into this category, and so does chicken. I have heard the warning enough times that eating duck and lamb can prolong the healing of wounds to be willing to stay away from them, and I do believe that most chicken sold in supermarkets these days carry too much growth hormone to be good for cancer patients.

I do not know if these warnings are valid. One thing I know for sure – my friends do not know either, nor do they understand why or how "re" or "du" works. Their friendly culinary advice was a mixed bag of hearsay, tradition, and folk medicine sprinkled with a bit of science or pseudo-science. I found such advice from my peers amusing because many saw themselves as Westernized, sometimes even speaking derisively of Chinese traditional practices, yet they clung to these beliefs and dished out such advice for me. Neither East nor West! And I am no better.

After hearing their advice a few times, I began to wonder if I would be left with any meat to eat were I to take what they said seriously. No beef, no chicken, no lamb, no duck! Would I turn vegetarian? Or vegan? I would not have much protein if I did that. Epiphany! Pork, of course! The only remaining meat, and a popular one in the Chinese diet!

The province of Guangdong in southeastern China is renowned for its culinary sophistication. Their chefs have the penchant to turn everything inhabiting the planet earth into tasty food for the table. The suspected origin of SARS or the Covid pandemic from civet cat and other animals in the wild have dented the enthusiasm for these exotic dishes, but old habits die hard. To this day a visit to some restaurants in Guangzhou, the provincial capital, and other smaller cities in the province will likely confirm this observation. The shop fronts of some of these eating places may not be as confusing as the wet markets one sees on television, and their displays are more orderly; nevertheless, it is possible for someone not familiar with the culture to mistake a restaurant with creepy crawly or jumpy creatures in cages at the entrance for a pet shop or another displaying animal innards in large bottles as a laboratory showing off its specimens. I will not elaborate or itemize these living creatures or the organs; doing that can easily turn Western readers off and upset their stomachs. To be fair, these Guangdong chefs have an ingenious way of transforming the ingredients into tasty delicacies, and some adventurous Westerners ready to try new foods have enjoyed them so long as they do not know what they are eating.

Most of my friends were born in Hong Kong but their parents or grandparents had come from Guangdong and brought with them their culinary traditions and secret recipes. They passed these on to their progeny, and my friends shared with me their secret family formulae on cooking pork. They told me to avoid the "grease and smoke" of frying. I can accept that; cooking in high heat produces heterocyclic amines (HCA) in meat that can increase the chance of getting cancer. They recommended boiling or steaming; food cooked in these ways may not be tasty but is certainly healthier. They reminded me to use the shank. I never tried that before. When I did, I found the meat lean with little fat and tender even after being boiled for a long time. One friend said I was to boil pork with an apple; another suggested adding pear with almonds. The recipes got more complicated and elaborate as times went by. I was to cook pork shank with lotus seed, red dates, barley, and large almonds; another suggested pork with yam and wolfberries. The ingredients to be added to the stew became more exotic – boil pork with the medicinal herbs bei qi (astragalus membrane) and dang shen (condonopsis roots). Another suggested adding ganoderma lucidum, the famous oriental mushrooms and elixir to give immortality to nobles and emperors of the distant past.

I did not know what these ingredients were good for, if they worked, or how they worked, but I followed their advice just the same when I could lay my hands on them. I had nothing to lose. Consuming those foods, especially in small amounts, would not kill me. Chinese have been taking these for centuries; they have survived and increased in number to make China one of the most populous countries in the world. I asked my husband Victor to get the ingredients at the local Chinese stores.

In a city with few Chinese and no Chinatown, not all the recommended ingredients were available in the handful of ethnic grocery stores in town. I did not have to worry. My friends recognized the challenge without my mentioning it. Not only did they send recipes; some bought what was needed, packaged it, and posted it to me. Soon I was receiving a steady supply in the mail. Two friends, one from San Francisco and another from Toronto, hand delivered the packages; they claimed to be passing through town, which was of course not the case. I understood, and I appreciated their visits.

I took the culinary advice and made some modifications. I did not always cook pork shank with the suggested ingredients or follow all the cooking instructions. Some ingredients were out of reach. At times I boiled the shank with vegetables instead; at other times I dumped the ingredients all together and all at once into the slow cooker to make soup, stew, or whatever you would call the medley that came out. Pork shank was the house specialty during the difficult months of cancer treatment. Pork shank soup and stew became the appetizer, soup, main course, and dessert for lunch and dinner. The same pot was not for the one meal; more often than not it was for the two meals of the day and sometimes for the next day and the day after until it was finished. When I did not have the appetite to eat what was before me, I broke the content into smithereens with a hand-held blender and gulped it down. I could not tell if these concoctions provided adequate nutrition to facilitate my recovery; I did not lose weight, and Victor, sharing the same fare, gained a few pounds.

Some friends also suggested juicing vegetables in the morning. These friends sent recipes too – three stalks of asparagus, four Brussels sprouts, two stalks of celery, a carrot, and more. I was not enamored with these ingredients. My mother had told me eating raw food would give me diarrhea; her early warning stuck, and I continue to heed it after all these years. I stay away from raw vegetables and salads. When Caucasian friends expressed surprise to see me skip salad in full-course meals, I usually said, "I am Chinese; I eat only cooked vegetables." This is a half-truth because Chinese do eat raw vegetables; only this one does not. When I received the juicing advice, I figured the vegetables would give me Vitamin C to boost immunity; fruits would bring the same benefits. Like what I did earlier, I modified their prophylactic advice and substituted vegetables with fruits, which in my opinion is equally nutritious and tastes a lot better.

My friends were not living in town, but I had their support just the same. They did not use any new technology to overcome the distance barrier; they did it the old-fashioned way. They called me regularly on the phone to see how I was doing, sent me packages of food by post to speed my recovery, one drove for miles to bring me food, and another flew in with the package to visit me. Quite a few friends my age had given up driving; those who continued driving often stayed within the neighborhood, not venturing far. We were no longer as mobile or adventurous as we used to be. Even if we were living in the same city, we would not see each other very often. Nevertheless, my friends did what they could from afar to give me emotional support and tangible help; we could not have been closer.

In any social interaction, kinks and problems can emerge; this happens in the closest and smoothest of relationships.

I appreciated and was grateful for my friends' help; however, sometimes I got upset with their attempts to do so. We might be far apart, hundreds of miles from each other, but I still felt at times their expressions of concern suffocating, or to put it bluntly, too authoritative for my taste.

Chinese respect and obey their elders. This tradition may have been diluted over time, but when seniors speak, juniors still listen; when the former gives a directive, the latter follows or is expected to follow. At this ripe old age, my friends and I joined ranks with these venerable elders. Victor and I have no children; we cannot enjoy the perks that come with aging. Friends who had children exercised their privileges; these matriarchs and patriarchs spoke with authority to their children and grandchildren; some got so used to it they did the same to me. After giving me advice on my diet, a retired elementary schoolteacher friend told me in the authoritative, patronizing voice she once used with her students, then on her children and grandchildren and now on me, "Now you know how to do it; do it." I did not like being told what to do, particularly in the way she said it. In the past, I might jokingly remind her we were peers or tell her she was clinging too long to her teaching habits. In my illness, it seemed I lost the inclination to do that and the ability to make my point casually. I did not say anything; I only stewed.

Other Chinese friends called to see if I followed their culinary instructions.

"Have you been juicing?" one asked over the phone. She had given me the suggestion and sent the recipes.

"It is hard work," I replied.

I was doing it religiously every day; I did not tell her that and I do not know why. Juicing was onerous work at the time; that was the first thought that came to mind when she asked, and I blurted it out. If I had told her what I had been doing, I would gain some brownie points and be spared from what followed. The spontaneous answer gave the impression I was neglectful; I was in for harsh words.

"I shopped for organic vegetables and did it every morning when Edward had cancer. Juicing is easy and takes no time."

She said this disapprovingly, forgetting that she was not the one afflicted with cancer, her husband, Edward, was. Here, the juicer and patient were one. I should have said something, but again, sickness took away my inclination and ability to speak up for myself. In better and, to be accurate, in healthier times I would have corrected myself and told her I was doing it every day. If I was in a bad mood, I would tell her off, and if I did not, it was because I deemed her remark unworthy of a response. Even when I took umbrage at being accused of insubordination and sloth with no basis, I kept quiet, I did not say anything, and I stewed. I was upset enough to tell Victor. He told me the remarks were meant as an encouragement. Like my attempt to comfort Juanita, his explanation did not work, and I was not appeased.

Father was cheerful to the last days of his life. He had a big smile for my friends when he ran into them on the street. They told me time and time again that his voice sounded strong, implying he was in exceptionally good health for someone of his age. I did not say anything to the contrary because Father would not want me to broadcast what he was going through. I followed his example when I had cancer and did not mention my discomforts. My friends made the same remark about me as they did with my father. More than once I was told, "Your voice is strong; you're all right." Others asked me what I did to kill time not realizing I had the energy to do only the bare minimum; one even invited herself to be my houseguest over Christmas, perhaps to keep me company. I flatly turned her down.

I was not disturbed when friends commented on how strong my father looked; I was proud. When they made similar comments about me, I was upset and offended. I felt they were making light of my discomforts, minimizing if not denying me my sick status and coming close to accusing me of faking cancer when it was I who put up a strong front in the first place. I knew they did not mean it that way, but I was upset. I did not know why. I reacted to their remarks in the same negative way as I did with my friends' untoward comments on my sloth and insubordination; I did not speak my mind, and I did not tell them how I felt.

I was not myself during my illness. I was sensitive, if not hypersensitive, interpreting, misinterpreting, and reinterpreting what friends said and more often than not adding a dark patina to what I had heard. I was less tolerant, less understanding, and less reasonable. I was turned off by the most innocuous statement, got upset with innocent remarks, was offended by the slightest negative comment, and took issue with what was said even when the words were not meant that way. And worse, I lost the ability to speak my mind. I did not say anything, I did not explain myself, and I did not take any action to correct the situation.

I kept the negative feelings inside, I fumed, and I stewed. This was not the usual way I reacted to anything upsetting me; it was unhealthy. The passivity was not pacificity. I vented the frustrations in other ways and on other people. I became unresponsive to encouragement and rejected offers of help. At times I was sullen and grouchy. On the odd occasion I could be abrasive and abusive, lashing out at anyone who happened to be around, and more than likely I did it to those who really cared for me and stayed around.

Being ill did not give me license to behave like that. I was bad. I can only imagine what those around me had to take and am grateful for their patience and tolerance. Many friends took my nonsense over the phone, and poor Victor took it in person every time, every day. They cared for me enough to ignore my uncalled-for and unforgivable behavior and did not abandon me. Instead, they reciprocated the bad behavior with understanding and support. They listened quietly to my complaints, acknowledged my problems, corrected my convoluted thinking, tolerated my irrational behavior, and ever so gently steered me away from the pit I was digging to bury myself.

After going through an emotional roller coaster on this cancer journey, I can only tell myself never to do it if I should become a patient again. I keep my fingers crossed that breast cancer will never come again; if it does, I will not repeat my bad behavior. And if I am a caregiver, I have to be equally sensitive, equally considerate, and equally appreciative of what the sick person is going through as my friends and Victor have been to relieve the patient's pain, be it physical or emotional.

EIGHT

Bills to Pay

The office of Dr. Gold, the medical oncologist, was not far from Grace Hospital where I had surgery. It was located in the city's medical district with a dozen or more medical plazas clustered together within a three-mile radius. One could find doctors in almost every specialty of medicine, from neurology to podiatry, neurosurgery to psychiatry, orthopedics to dermatology, pediatrics to geriatrics, gynecology to urology, cardiology to physical therapy, outpatient surgery to pain management, and many more. If one needed prompt attention, aside from the emergency room of Grace Hospital, there were clinics offering urgent care and walk-in consultation. One could find healthcare for almost every ailment in every stage of a disease in the vicinity.

The medical oncologist's clinic was in a plaza on a quiet street a little way from the busy traffic of the main drag. The plaza was long and narrow, too small to provide the space or too new to give time for trees to grow; only rosemary shrubs marked the entrances at the two ends. Two rows of flat-roofed adobe-like buildings lined the narrow driveway threading through the mall, and the monotony of their earth-tone façade was punctuated by the red tiles on the eaves to provide shade for pedestrians. The doctor's office was the first or the last unit of the inner row depending on which end one entered the plaza. Dr. Gold's name, together with five other hematologists, was etched in bold black letters on the glass panel adjacent to the front entrance.

His assistant had turned me away earlier because I did not have the second pathology report. As soon as I obtained one from Dr. Shield, I called the oncologist's office to get an appointment. Dr. Gold reminded me of the surgeon, equally serious and reserved, a bit older, a bit taller, and a bit fairer. He moved fast in the hallway with his long white medical coat hanging loosely from his slightly hunched shoulders and flapping vigorously in sync as he walked from one examination room to the next. His brisk gait together with his knitted brows gave the impression of a busy man deep in thought.

I was doing something right following medical protocol when I met with this doctor to look at the results of the pathology report that came out after surgery to decide on the next course of treatment. I faxed Dr. Gold a copy in case Dr. Shield did not send it to him and I took one with me to the meeting. The medical oncologist never received anything; I showed him the copy I brought. The doctor mustered a smile after going over the content. It was easy for a doctor to tell the patient the prognosis when she had stage 1 breast cancer; he would have a more difficult time breaking the news to those in advanced stages of the disease.

I gave Dr. Gold a rundown of the treatment received so far and the arrangements made for further treatment – surgery done and radiation scheduled; in return he asked me a few questions on my family medical history. Since I had made arrangements for radiation, he told me he would order a blood test to see if I would need additional chemotherapy. He was referring to the ONCOtype DX test to check if I carried the gene predisposing me to breast cancer. Angelina Jolie had her double mastectomy for that reason, and others carrying the genes may undergo chemotherapy as a safeguard even with early-stage breast cancer.

Dr. Gold and his colleagues ran a center on the premise offering patients chemotherapy – an infusion of a concoction of different drugs to "cure" cancer. I did not know what went on behind the closed doors of the section offering chemotherapy treatment; it was all quiet in the waiting area. There was no small talk among the patients one sometimes encountered in medical waiting rooms; no one violated the very visible interdict to speak on cell phones, making the notice on the wall superfluous. The pale faces, bald heads, drawn looks, and the shriveled bodies slouched in the seats or strapped to the wheelchairs told me these patients had little desire or energy to break the rule. What I saw that afternoon confirmed my readings on the web on the deleterious and debilitating side effects of chemotherapy and strengthened my resolve to avoid it at all costs. The doctor's wait-and-see strategy was more than fine with me.

Three days before I was to go over the blood test results with the doctor, a woman called me at home.

"This is … from the True Light Test Company. You did a blood test with us."

"Yes?" The word was more a query on what was to follow than an affirmative answer to the question if there was one.

"You have to pay before we can release the result," the woman said.

Her voice was not intimidating, but the threat was unmistakable. Could release? Or would release? It did not matter. The message was the same – she would withhold valuable information from me unless money changed hands.

"How much is the bill?"

"Two thousand."

I almost fell off the chair. I had paid $10–20 for blood tests, and on the rare occasion $100, but never $2,000. The number was high. It shocked me out of my cancer brain fog. How would I know she was not an imposter? How would I know if she really represented the company? She could be a fraud who happened to know I took the blood test; it could be a scam. The number displayed on the phone told me the call was from Florida. Dr. Gold and his nurse never mentioned the location of the testing company. If the company was in Florida, there was no way to verify if the call came from the outfit; even a number the same as the testing company could be fake, masquerading as the legitimate one. Con artists can use computers to play any trick. I did not give the caller my credit card number as she had requested; I asked for the address to send a check with no intention to follow through before talking with Dr. Gold.

Her request made me think of funeral homes bilking griev-
ing families – some dishonest establishments take advantage of the bereaved to overcharge or sell them services they
do not need. How many have the experience in these matters, know much about funeral arrangements, or are familiar with the going rates? Most do not. These families are
too distraught to be in a position to find the best provider
or to negotiate for the best price; they usually accept what
these establishments recommend and pay what is asked.
Cancer patients seeking treatment are in a not-too-different
situation. My cancer might not be life-threatening, but I still
felt the urgency to do something about it as soon as possible, and I jumped at the first treatment offer. I knew nothing about cancer treatment or treatment protocol let alone
the costs. I did not shop around for the "best" treatment,
the "best" doctor, or the "best" price for the services. Had I
wanted to get the information I would not know where to
begin; neither did I have the energy nor the mood to do it. I
took whatever came my way.

Victor and I were frugal and careful with money. When it
came to a question of paying medical bills to save my life,
the answer was clear – we would do everything within our
means. We would not consider cost; we would pay whatever
the providers asked so long as we had the resources, and we
would empty our life savings for this purpose if needed.
The demand for payment in medical treatment worked
almost like a ransom; I was ready and more than willing
to give anything, especially when the provider threatened
to withhold services. I held back only because I wanted to
verify if she really represented the company.

I told Dr. Gold about the phone call and warned him he might not have the test results because I had not paid, and I was right. Dr. Gold said he would look into it and left the room. I waited more than fifteen minutes; for once I was happy to wait because I could imagine what he was doing. He came back with three sheets of paper and went over the findings with me. He said I would gain little with additional chemotherapy and that he would not recommend it; I was relieved. However, he told me I had to come back after I finished radiation. He did not tell me why, and I did not ask. The web doctor, however, told me Dr. Gold would prescribe me adjuvant treatment to prevent cancer from recurring. The medical oncologist never mentioned the bill for the blood test and the woman never called again.

In September 2014 national television stations reported that Farid Fata, a hematologist-oncologist, was charged with $35 million in overbilling. According to these reports he prescribed chemotherapy to patients longer than necessary, gave it to others who would not benefit from it, and worse, to others who did not have cancer! The patients suffered health damages, and a few died. It would be hard to tell if the victims died from the treatment or from cancer, but it was clear this doctor did not have the patients' interests at heart. Who would not believe a doctor telling them they had cancer? I never questioned Dr. Gray. Who would not panic when they learned they had cancer? I did. And who would not follow the doctor's orders in the situation? I did without hesitation, doing what the doctors told me. Patients trust doctors and follow their instructions; it is easy to take advantage of patients under such circumstances. Fata was found guilty, forfeited $17.6 million, and received a forty-five-year prison sentence. His patients received some justice, but the harm was done. They would never get back their health and suffer irreparable health damages from the unnecessary toxin. Now that I had joined the ranks of cancer patients, I felt especially for these victims.

I am happy that Dr. Gold was not that type. I would not have known if he had given me the same unnecessary treatment; if he did I would take it without question and follow his instructions. He did not do that; he did not prescribe me chemotherapy, and more than likely he negotiated with the blood test company to get the results. Months later I got a bill from the company amounting to about 5 per cent of what was asked.

When Dr. Gold's nurse checked my vitals in the examination room, I told her about the payment call. She said that the healthcare provider should settle the bill with the insurance company before approaching the client for the portion not covered; the woman from the blood test company should not have called me. She advised me to hold off paying until I received the bill in the mail. How many patients would know how these things work? I didn't.

In my experience, things never happened that way. Health service providers almost always demanded payment before the delivery of service. They usually called a few days prior to the scheduled procedure asking me to bring a credit card, cash, or a certified check of a specified amount when I came for the appointment. I always did as I was told, never raising any questions. Even after talking with Dr. Gold's nurse, I did the same. I did not have the energy to fight or the courage to defy the service providers lest the service needed would be withheld. I paid close to $1,000 for the surgery and $6,000 for radiation prior to receiving the treatment procedure. At least I was paying the bona fide service providers.

I do not condone their behavior, but I can see the reasoning behind the action. Money in hand is better than what comes later, and there is no guarantee that the clients who have received the service will pay. They protect themselves by making sure the cost or part of the cost is covered; what better time to do it than just prior to the delivery of services! Making the demand at this time carries the threat of withholding service if money is not paid; it is hard for patients to ignore the request because they may go without the treatment they need or want. And these amounts are usually much higher than the co-pays; to be fair, the providers refund the overpaid amount to the clients, though at a much later date.

I was lucky to be able to pay these bills. I could not help wondering what would happen if I could not. These were not small sums; some might not be able to afford it, and others might be unable to come up with the money at such short notice. What would happen if I could not pay the bill? Was there any way I could have not paid and received treatment? Or paid less? Even if I could pay at this point, I could not help thinking the medical bills piling up from a long, drawn-out illness could leave me penniless. Would I be reduced to living in poverty or on social assistance? Being ill is bad enough, and to be reduced to penury paying medical bills is worse. It could have happened to me, and it could happen to anyone in the circumstances.

I had health insurance coverage, a steady pension, and enough savings to cover the unexpected expenses; otherwise, the medical bills for stage 1 breast cancer would have pulled me into a hole. If I could not pay, would I have had to forego surgery or radiation? If this were the case, the cancer could or would spread and I might die from it. It would be a death sentence, albeit a deferred one. From what I gathered, to suffer through the last stage of the disease without morphine or other such opioids to alleviate the discomfort is excruciatingly painful. Even if cancer remained localized and did not spread, I would be living in constant fear.

When the economy tanked in 2008, two friends with diabetes lost their jobs and health insurance. One took less insulin each time or less frequently to stretch it out over a longer period of time; I do not know exactly what he did, but it was something like that. Another stopped taking it altogether when she ran out of money. Doing that did not kill them; their quality of life in the years to come, however, was heavily compromised as a result. One lost two toes and the other, her sight. In my cancer support group, a woman left for Mexico because the same treatment cost less than $1,000, a fraction of what it would cost her in the States. When I questioned the quality of the drug she would be getting, she told me it was not something she would consider because getting some treatment was better than receiving none. Another member in the support group postponed a PET scan for her metastasizing brain tumor because she could not afford the procedure. Without the resources, her only option was to go without it. These are sad stories I would like to forget. Both stopped coming to the meeting soon after, and I never learned the outcome of their action. I could only wish them well.

I have always thought that healthcare, like education, is a citizen's God-given right, especially in an affluent country like the United States; it appears not to be the case. My diabetic friends and cancer support group comrades were honest, working people who did not have adequate resources to cover their medical bills through no fault of their own. They had to forego essential treatment they could not afford only to suffer disastrous fallouts that maimed them for life, and I have other friends under similar circumstances being totally drained of their resources by paying medical bills. True, the government comes in to help the destitute and penniless but not those with any tangible assets. It is only after these hardworking people have exhausted all their resources before they can get Medicaid or other help. It is a stressful and humiliating experience to get these types of government assistance; no one wants to go through that.

Advocates of a private healthcare system emphasize the importance of freedom and personal choice, with patients going wherever, to whomever, and whenever they want to seek medical help. This freedom and choice are nice if one can afford it. For those without adequate resources, getting needed medical help is the issue, not the choice of whom to see or where to go. The latter is a luxury beyond their reach. Indeed, in the case of cancer, the American Cancer Society has pointed out that having the financial resources for treatment is a better predictor of survival than the stage of the disease. Money talks in matters of health.

What happened to my friends and the two members of my cancer support group got me thinking about how lucky Father was in Hong Kong. The government doctors were courteous and competent, as good as those in private practice, and the government facilities were equal to if not better than many private ones. He received checkups every three months and timely treatment once a problem was diagnosed. A visit to the clinic cost about US$5 charged as a registration fee, which also covered consultation and drugs to last until the next appointment. And when he stayed in the hospital, he paid about US$15 a day for the bed he occupied, food, the doctor's consultation fee, the operation if one was performed, and whatever else was needed. The charges will have gone up since then, but it would still be very affordable to the general public. Those with money use private medical services. The cost is much higher, and the prices vary widely; a day's hospital stay can range from US$200 for a bed to over US$2,000 for a private room with the additional charges for meals, antiseptics, and other items commensurate with the type of accommodation chosen; the more expensive the accommodation, the more costly the other items. Canada has public healthcare. The provision of medical care in some provinces is funded entirely through taxes; and in others, citizens pay the government small insurance premiums, nothing like the hefty ones in the States. When Canadians see their doctors or stay in the hospital, the patients pay nothing and the government reimburses the healthcare providers. I paid thousands of dollars before I could get cancer treatment, even with insurance coverage.

Contrary to the popular belief that cancer patients wait a long time before getting medical help in a publicly funded system, this seems not to be the case. True, it may take some time before one gets a medical test in Hong Kong or Canada; once cancer is diagnosed, treatment follows quickly. The Hong Kong government estimates that these patients receive treatment within two months after being diagnosed. In Canada, oncologists are to see new cancer patients within two weeks of referral; I do not know if there is a similar mandated timeline for patients to receive treatment. My information is anecdotal. A Canadian friend received treatment two weeks after her diagnosis of breast cancer; another received surgery within the month. I would have to wait three weeks to see the surgeon Dr. Gray initially recommended and longer before the tumor would be taken out if I had not switched to Dr. Shield.

I am grateful to have insurance coverage and enough savings to cover the medical expenses, at least in this round of cancer treatment, but I cannot help feeling envious of my friends with their socialized medical care. My Hong Kong friends using the public healthcare system for the same treatment would have spent a couple hundred American dollars and my Canadian ones not a dime; I had to pay much more even with insurance coverage. For five years after the active treatment phase breast cancer patients take preventive drugs to keep the cancer from coming back. My Canadian friends paid nothing or next to nothing, and I paid $100 every three months to get the same drug. It is simply hard for me to understand how a rich country like the United States cannot provide its citizens similar benefits.

NINE

Radiation

The radiation clinic was an impressive stand-alone building with its own parking lot, nothing like the crammed offices in medical buildings with insufficient or nonexistent parking space that I was accustomed to. The lobby was an eye-opener; it had a coffee machine, a hot water dispenser, teabags, cream, and sugar for patients to make themselves a cup of coffee or tea – something I have never seen in a medical office. When I started radiation and went beyond the reception area I saw more offices, examination rooms, changing rooms, and the big treatment room with its radiation equipment in the rear.

I like women breaking barriers and moving into prestigious careers once dominated by men and was happy to have Dr. McEwan, a female doctor, looking after me. She was in her late forties or perhaps early fifties. She graduated from a good medical school on the West Coast and spent her residency at an equally renowned cancer institute nearby. She came across as the typical professional woman, articulate, confident, capable, and she lived up to my stereotypical image of redheads, ebullient, effusive, and effervescent. Her bubbly personality was contagious and put patients at ease. I am not the sociable type; I do not know how she got me talking about the restaurants in town, almost forgetting what brought me to her office.

The doctor gave me and Victor a ten-minute expose on radiation and treatment – a much livelier and more engaging presentation than the other two doctors looking after my care. Radiation kills cancer cells at the primary site and any vagrant ones that may have wandered away to the surrounding tissues. She suggested two ways to do it – conventional X-ray radiation or hypofractionation. She said the latter was a newer procedure than the first involving fewer sessions with a stronger dosage each time but equally safe and producing similar if not better results. Victor and I were all for efficacy and efficiency, but we were cautious. Victor reasoned that the conventional time-tested method of delivering a smaller dosage each time would be safer than hypofractionation; less damage would be done if a mistake was made. I went along with his safety concern and picked the latter.

Radiation kills cancer cells with beams of intense energy. Different types of beams are used to treat cancers located in different parts of the body. For example, electron beams are used to treat the skin and tumors close to the surface, and photon beams or X-rays are used in breast cancer. These different beams are delivered in three main ways – external, internal, and systemic. As these terms suggest, in the case of external radiation beams come from an outside source;

in internal radiation or brachytherapy, radioactive materials are placed at the target site to be taken out later and in some cases remain in the body after its radioactivity is spent; and with systemic radiation the radioactive materials are injected into the body, circulate in the bloodstream, and expelled through sweating or urination.

I had conventional X-ray radiation for breast cancer treatment. The X-ray comes from an outside source. Electrons traveling at high velocity in the accelerator hit a metal target such as tungsten to generate photons. Photons fan out like the headlight of a car and a collimator with wedges and blocks aligns, directs, and focuses the beam to its target; and in my case, the tumor bed in the breast. The high-energy beam penetrates tissues, disrupts the molecular bonds of the DNA in cancer cells, kills the cells, and stops them from reproducing. Hypofractionation, the "newer procedure" the doctor recommended, also uses external X-rays; but the number of radiation sessions is fewer, with a higher dose each time.

On this first visit Dr. McEwan told me to come back for radiation a month after surgery. I was happy with the arrangement. The surgeon would take out the tumor and radiation would clean up any vagrant malignant cells that might have escaped into the surrounding tissues and I would be rid of cancer in no time! Little did I know I was jumping the gun to schedule radiation with the tumor not removed.

The incision appeared closed in four weeks, and I went to see Dr. McEwan. She declared me ready for radiation and explained the treatment logistics – "preparation" of the breast for the procedure the coming Monday, radiation simulation on Friday, and radiation to start on the Monday after. I would be irradiated five days a week; the number of radiation sessions went up from the twenty she mentioned at the earlier meeting to thirty-three, the highest number of sessions a breast cancer patient usually gets, perhaps also an indication of the maximum radiation dose a patient can safely take.

I was not thinking of these upper limits at the time; I was curious about the jump in the number of radiation sessions. However, I did not ask the doctor. The habitual restrain to ask questions might have come from my upbringing, but it was certainly reinforced by the medical doctors' behavior. Years ago, allergies suddenly flared up one spring, giving me a runny nose and causing me to sneeze. I never had this before, and I was curious to know why; I asked more questions than the doctor in the student clinic cared to answer. He gave a cursory response to the first question; when I followed with a second, he showed his annoyance in no uncertain terms.

"You do not trust me," he said.

I did not mean it that way at all. I was not questioning his expertise; I only wanted to understand why I had allergies all of a sudden. He did not see it that way and interpreted my questions as a sign of mistrust or a challenge to his authority and was offended. The message was clear – patients were not supposed to ask doctors questions. This was not the first or the last time something like this happened; many doctors had brushed aside my questions, but none had put it as bluntly as he did. I learned my lesson from these incidences – doctors wanted silent acquiescence from patients.

I had not read about the doctors' signal for patients to leave in Dr. Marsh's *Do No Harm*, but I sensed as much when Dr. McEwan asked me if I had any questions. She uncrossed her legs, planted her feet on the floor, and bent her torso a little forward – preparatory moves to get up from the chair. I wanted to ask her about the increased number of radiation sessions, but I knew this would delay her leaving and would not be appreciated. Besides, she might interpret my curiosity as second-guessing her and would be offended. It would do a patient no good to be on the wrong side with the doctor looking after her. I left the question unasked and unanswered.

"Preparing" the breast for radiation involves two steps: first, taking a CT scan to provide a three-dimensional image of the breast and, second, marking the surface of the chest for the administration of radiation.

On Monday the nurse at the radiation clinic injected me with a shot of dye to sharpen the contrast in the images taken by the CT scanner. She warned me I would feel flushed. I did not know what "feeling flushed" meant; as usual I kept the query to myself, this time to cover my ignorance of the English language. After a short wait I was ushered into the room for the procedure. The huge arch of the scanner reminded me of a large half donut with a table/bed under it. I climbed onto the table and lay perfectly still; the bed moved slowly forward until the arch was directly over my breast. I saw no flashes and heard no clicks from the shutters as the machine quietly took multiple pictures. In the middle of it all, I felt like peeing. It dawned on me what the polite euphemism "feeling flushed" meant. I was grateful the nurse warned me it was a false sensation. I did not panic and the urgency went away after a while.

Next, I found myself lying bare-chested on an examination table in another room with a stranger looking down at me. By this time, I was so used to stripping that I was quick to do it when asked and did not feel embarrassed at all doing it in front of a man or woman, stranger or not. This not-too-tall Indian fellow staring down at my bare chest did not disturb me one bit. He had to be an American of East Indian origin. His brown skin, black curly hair, and dark brown eyes with long lashes betrayed his East Indian ancestry, and his accent suggested he was brought up if not born in the States. He told me politely he would mark my breast to facilitate the X-rays targeting the tumor. He belonged to the rare breed of medical personnel to explain to patients what they are about to do.

My chest became his canvas. He used his marker to draw grid lines on my right breast and made a huge asterisk, probably where the tumor was located or perhaps where the X-rays were to go in. He protected the best part of his handiwork, the asterisk, with a transparent tape. His next move, however, took me off guard; he told me he would tattoo three points below the rib cage. It had never occurred to me to get one and I had not even pierced my ears; I saw such action rightly or wrongly as self-mutilation that might be painful and would not add to my looks. In any case, tattooing was a young people's fad, not for someone at my age. Now it was a requirement in a medical procedure, not a decision for me to make. The process was short and painless; the tattoo was there before I knew it was done, and the three marks stay to this day.

After finishing his artistic creation this man told me he would take pictures of my breast. The pictures were for the medical physicist and dosimetrist who would calculate the strength and angle of the beam to target the tumor bed in the breast. He would not have bothered me if he had said he wanted to get it as a souvenir of his handy artwork. What followed was a surprise. He took out his cell phone, not a camera, to snap the shots. Young people take selfies and pictures of food with their smartphones; it never occurred to me to use it to take pictures of my breast! So a smartphone is more than a toy or accessory; it is a piece of equipment used in medical procedures too!

Friday was the radiation dry run. I walked into the radiotherapy bunker, a place I would visit thirty-three times to receive radiation in the days to follow. True to the label "bunker," these places are carefully designed and solidly constructed to shield the employees and patients from unwanted damaging radiation. But unlike the plain, bare bunkers built for shelters, these are spacious and airy to accommodate the operation of the accelerator, to perform radiation treatment, and to make the patients feel comfortable and at ease. As a patient, I only had access to the treatment room; it was certainly very different from the operating room for my breast surgery and lived up to the medical treatment facility I had imagined.

The accelerator, with its collimator, stood against the wall in the sizable treatment room, a rectangular light beige console about the height of an adult person or perhaps a little taller with a huge arm jutting out at a right angle from one side. The end of the arm reminded me of the overhead light hanging from the ceiling of the operating room; only it emitted invisible X-rays, not the beams that would light up the place for the doctors to perform the operation. At the foot of the accelerator was a table for the patient to lie down to receive radiation.

The control room was a step up from the treatment room separated by a huge glass panel allowing the operators to see every movement below. It had an impressive array of panels, with switches and display screens on the long counter flushed against the divide. A television with its camera focused on the accelerator and treatment table was mounted from the ceiling a little behind the operator's seat so the person could monitor what was going on in the radiation room even with his or her back turned.

Ruby and John together ran the radiotherapy bunker. John was in his late thirties and, I assumed, the senior, and Ruby, in her twenties, was probably the junior of the team. They could be older; at my age everyone looked young. I would see these two radiation therapists five days a week for the next seven weeks, came to know them well, and liked them an awful lot.

Again, I found myself unabashedly stripped to the waist, lying on the treatment table. They asked me to turn my head to the left and have my left hand hold my right wrist, which was resting on the bed above my head. Together they shifted my torso this way and that, left and right, up and down, a little at a time. I did not know the reference points in the positioning, and most likely they used the grid points and tattoo marks painted on my chest. Ruby was left to do the fine tuning with all the required touching of my body while John stood by; he would probably take over the detailed adjustments if the patient was a man.

They left the room and Ruby's soothing voice came through the intercom assuring me they could hear me if I needed anything. Some patients might be anxious being left in the room alone waiting to be irradiated; I was not, or I believed I was not. Nevertheless, I found her calming voice perfectly suited for the occasion. Moments later the two returned to pull and push me a little more and left the bunker one more time for the control room. They seemed satisfied and Ruby announced I could leave.

Some clinics custom-make molds to cradle the patients so they will be in the same position in every radiation session; a friend undergoing twenty sessions for her breast cancer treatment on the East Coast was given one. I did not get any; the pushing and pulling were repeated when I returned on Monday, but the whole process took much less time than the first, and the positioning exercise was repeated in every session over the next seven weeks.

On Monday I had my first radiation session. When Ruby and John were satisfied with my position, they left the room. The door closed and the red light at the entrance blinked to warn people to stay away; I was the only one inside. Ruby's calming voice came through the intercom reminding me to stay still and assuring me once again she could hear me if I needed anything. The accelerator purred and stopped almost immediately.

"You are breathing fast. Are you all right?" Ruby's pellucid voice came through the speaker.

"I have a breathing problem. I have allergies," I answered.

I did have allergies, but the gasping was more than likely no different from the high blood pressure scores the nurse found prior to surgery – a physiological giveaway of the anxiety beneath my seemingly sedate exterior.

I was not the only patient to react that way; many before me were equally anxious and breathing just as fast. My reaction came as no surprise to John and Ruby; they had a ready solution. Ruby did not dispute my lame explanation and made a suggestion that I thought at the time was brilliant; I did not know it was a much-tested antidote suggested to many patients many times before. She said, "Stop breathing," and I held my breath. When the accelerator finished zapping, she said, "Breathe," and I would breathe normally.

To take my mind off when I was to stop breathing for the machine to send X-rays into my body, I started counting. "One, two, three, four … " I reached thirty when the machine stopped purring. When I told a friend I held my breath for a count of thirty, she marveled at how long I could go without air. She did not know I was rushing through the numbers at breakneck speed, counting in monosyllabic Cantonese, a Chinese dialect without the tonal nuances of English, which allowed me to squeeze in more numerals than I could have done otherwise in the same period of time.

When Ruby uttered the word "breathe" over the intercom, my belly muscles contracted to push out the dirty air through my nose as fast as possible, making a sound almost like a sigh. I gladly took in one slow, deep breath of fresh air, and it never felt so good. Then I inhaled and exhaled normally; this did not last long. The accelerator arm moved from the right to my left and Ruby said, "Stop breathing." I took in one deep breath, held it, began a second round of counting, and received a second round of zapping with the invisible photon beam penetrating my breast from a different angle.

From the new position of the accelerator arm I could see a row of red lights lining the rectangular lens at the end. The lights could not have been the X-rays that are supposedly invisible to the naked eye; they were more than likely lights to help align the X-rays to the target. At the thought I closed my eyes to keep the rays out, even though I knew full well it would be a futile precaution. If the X-rays hit my eyes, the beams that could penetrate breast tissues would certainly pierce my eyelids to reach my retina. I closed my eyes just the same and resumed counting in my native tongue. In less than fifteen minutes I was back in the changing room with the day's procedure over.

Since my diagnosis of breast cancer in September, my life had changed. The calendar did not follow the days of the week or the dates of the month but followed the schedule required for treatment. My daily activities involved and revolved around the efforts to rid me of cancer. First it was one test, then another, and more tests to be done before surgery. Surgery went smoothly and the incision closed. Phase two involved preparing for radiation and then the radiation itself. I finished the first session with thirty-two more to follow. From now on, weekdays would be radiation days, weekends would be breaks from the procedure; that would be the new routine. The treatment sessions would be over by the end of December, and I would likely see Dr. Gold, the medical oncologist, in January to start the third treatment phase. I could not and would not be able to see my father at Christmas as I had said I would; the trip to Hong Kong had to wait till mid-January at the earliest, if not later, and Father would be disappointed with another delay. There was no point telling him now; it would only upset him and make him worry. I would break the news to him when the time came closer, perhaps in early or mid-December.

TEN

Shopping Aerobics

Unlike some medical clinics where patients with appointments have to wait half an hour or more before seeing the doctor, I never had to do that at Dr. McEwan's clinic. Sometimes I walked straight in for the procedure after signing in; even if I had to wait, it would be no more than ten minutes and would not give me enough time to even make a cup of coffee and enjoy it. The radiation treatment plus the change of clothes would be about half an hour and sometimes a little less.

The clinic was at the opposite end of town from our home; it took forty minutes to get there using the highway and longer if I drove through the city streets. The traveling and the half an hour at the clinic would come close to three hours and my morning would be shot. It was not that I had anything urgent to take care of; it was only my compulsive nature to use time efficiently, whatever that word might mean. If I had to go all that distance and spend all that time on the road for a half-hour procedure, I might as well do something on the way to make the trip worthwhile.

There is a Galleria Mall in almost every city, and mine was no exception. It was on the route to the clinic and the biggest shopping center in town with anchors like Dillard's, Nordstrom, Macy's, JCPenney, and some smaller stores catering to every consumer need. Christmas was two months away; I was not thinking of holiday shopping. My family and circle of friends had long agreed not to send each other gifts we mostly did not need or could not use; doing that would mean spending money needlessly with only the stores to benefit and adding to the clutter we wanted to get rid of. Instead, we sent each other Christmas cards sometimes accompanied with a report on what had transpired in the last twelve months. With the coming of the digital age even that had changed; we emailed greetings or sent e-cards with photos and messages. I was not planning to do anything different this year.

I was looking for an enclosed area to exercise. The hospital where I had had the surgery recommended daily arm exercises and medical friends had encouraged me to do the same. I did that at home, but I had not been out for walks for the lack of energy and a fear of pollutants that might trigger allergic reactions. A month had gone by since I had the operation and my fatigue had lifted somewhat, so I figured it might be time to start doing something with my legs. A walk in the mall after the radiation session would be good, and Galleria Mall was the perfect place; the half-hour walk from one end of the plaza to the other and back would be just right, and there were benches to sit down on if I needed a rest. Doing one round in the mall together with the arm exercises at home would be a complete workout.

Living in a small city had its advantages. Traffic was not bad during rush hour compared to those in the larger urban centers, and with a 9:30 radiation appointment I avoided the peak morning traffic on the way out to the clinic. The mall would be open when I finished radiation treatment, and if I was a few minutes early the wait would not be long. I did not know at the time that the mall opened at eight in the morning during the holiday season and I would never have to wait. The timing was perfect.

Everything in the mall reminded shoppers that Christmas was near. Big white, silver, and gold stars hanging from the ceiling floated above in the east and west wings, and a Christmas tree stood tall, reaching the balustrade on the second floor in the central rotunda. A shiny red garland entwined the fir from the lowest bough to its pinnacle, and the branches were decked with glittery red, blue, and green baubles, glitzy ornaments, and twinkly lights. Every store reminded customers of the holiday season selling them wares they were not to do without; as if these stores were not offering customers enough choices, makeshift stands sprang up in the once open space of the arcade pushing more of the same to passersby. And of course no one could miss good old Santa's studio where he would take pictures with children; only I was there too early to meet him in person.

Just as I did not like to play sick and continued with the domestic chores when I got news of my breast cancer, I turned down Victor's offer to give me a lift to the radiation clinic. I wanted to do things on my own after surgery when I had little energy and performing every task was a struggle; I was all the more determined to be self-reliant now that I was a little stronger. Making the daily journey would not be easy, but I would have the satisfaction of doing it myself and being independent. Besides, I intended to walk in the mall after radiation, and Victor has never liked shopping or shopping malls; he has always been reluctant to come along when I invite him. If I took him up on his offer, he would have to wait for me in the clinic and would be totally bored in the mall. He had done more than enough for me in the last month and more. I did not want to add another distasteful task for him.

My debilitated right arm was strong enough to downshift into Drive while my left hand remained on the wheel; I could drive. But it was too weak to up-shift from Drive to Reverse. Like putting dishes on the kitchen shelf, my left hand could support my right elbow to shift gears, but this would leave the wheel unattended. This would be a problem when I had to put the transmission into reverse, for example, to back out of a parking spot. My solution was simple – avoid the situation. I looked for single-row parking where I could drive in to park and drive ahead again to leave. Parking at the radiation clinic was spacious, and I was in the Galleria Mall early enough to find this type of space. I could not imagine what would happen if I suddenly had to go into reverse or, worse, got caught by the police with my physical handicap. I did not run into such a mishap. Being able to get away with it seemed an added adventure.

"Mall walk" was a new experience for me but not for many others; there were quite a few regulars doing it at this hour. It was not long before I could make out five familiar faces. They were my age or a bit younger and all looked fit as a fiddle with not an extra ounce of fat on their bodies. Two men did the walk together, so did two women; one woman, like me, did it solo. They wore gym outfits – sweatshirts, sweatpants, sneakers, with a bottle of water in hand or in a pouch strapped around their waist. I wore loose-fitting clothes that were easy to put on and take off for radiation, and my bottle of water stayed in the car, too heavy for me to carry the whole time. Before long we recognized and acknowledged one another; it was too late in the day to say good morning, so we nodded and smiled when passing each other.

I entered Macy's from the parking lot, went straight down the aisle and out of the department store, into the arcade, past the boutiques in the east wing, the central rotunda, more shops in the west wing, and into JCPenney until I reached its exit to the parking lot at the other end of the plaza; then I retraced my steps till I was back to the Macy's parking lot entrance, now my exit to get to the car. The mall-walking men took the same route I did. They marched down the aisle oblivious of what was displayed on the two sides; more often than not, they were deep in conversation. I overheard them more than once discussing the stock prices of the day and sometimes the scores of yesterday's football game. The two women did not say a word to each other; they moved in sync, stopped at the Macy's mall entrance, turned, and doubled back till they reached the entrance of JCPenney, stopped, made a 180-degree turn, and retraced their steps. I did not know how many rounds they did each day; it had to be more than one because I ran into them a few times doing my one-round walk. I was curious as to why they would not take the extra steps to go inside the department stores when it would add some distance to their walk. Looking back, I realized they were smart – they did not expose themselves to the temptations inside. This walking, shopping neophyte did not know better and walked straight into the stores, or should I say, the shopping traps.

I am not fashion-conscious. I need little and buy little. I often brag that my wardrobe is classic, standing the test of time, which really means I am not "in" with fashion. I have been wearing the same dowdy outfit, year in year out. Perhaps I have been discouraged to do anything different by my colleagues, almost all of them men; to dress up would be a violation of the dress code. They wore shirts and trousers with no tie or jacket, and a few went into the classroom in jeans; I fit well with this working crowd and I wore blouses and slacks for work. Whenever I put on a dress, something new, or something more proper for a faculty or university-level meeting, someone would inevitably query, "What's going on today?" I seldom went shopping and would go only when I needed something. These trips of necessity, however, did not stop me from buying things I fancied but might not need or might not use; I was especially vulnerable if a sale was on. When I brought the items home Victor would inevitably comment, "It must be on sale." He knows me all too well. And I would put the new acquisition away at the back of the closet and forget about it.

I walked the mall five days a week for about a month before I stopped. Those twenty-odd days of mall walking could certainly make up for the lost years when I stayed away from the shopping centers. Women's apparel was usually displayed on the second level of the department stores; it was not long before I switched my ground-floor route to walk upstairs. One round at that level would cover the ladies' sections of Macy's and JCPenney. Unlike the two women, I did not stop at the entrance and eagerly walked into the store. And unlike the men I could not keep my eyes straight on the path ahead; they swept like radars left and right. Soon I could tell where each kind of merchandise was displayed in each store, where the slacks were hung and the dresses were pinned high against the wall and where Michael Kors, Ralph Lauren, Perry Ellis, and other brands located their products. I could rattle off the prices of the items I liked, tell the number in stock, if they had been moved, and sometimes even how many were sold the day earlier. The stores could or should have made me their inventory clerk.

Retail stores do a third of their business around Christmas. They put on sales at this time of the year to attract customers – whether the advertised discounts translate into real savings for the consumer is another matter. In the first week of mall walking, I did not know better. Like an eagle zeroing in on its prey, I swooped down on the racks with big signs announcing 20 per cent discounts hung above them. I justified the detour to the rack like this: going over to take a look meant taking additional steps, adding up to a longer distance and more exercise for my legs. I circled the target rack, pounced on the article that caught my eye, grabbed my favorite color, and caressed it. If it was my size, the fitting room would be the next stop, giving me another opportunity to do more exercise with my arms and legs when I tried it on. If I was happy with it, the cashier's counter was the next destination. In the excitement, I forgot my lack of energy and fatigue, quickened my steps, made a beeline for the cashier, and claimed ownership of the prize.

I walked the mall early in the morning. The deluge of Christmas shoppers had not materialized, and there were no lines of customers waiting to pay. I finished the transaction in no time and felt lucky and happy. In those first weeks I brought home "bargains" I did not need and often would not use. Even today when I open the closet, I stare at clothes bought at the time that have never been and will never be worn. These purchases were usually not expensive; still, it was throwing away money I should not have spent.

Shopping daily was not only a novel experience; it gave me a lesson in retail sales and consumerism. Since I was not a seasoned shopper, I did not know how far and how quickly prices could drop. A 20 per cent discount seemed like a very good deal. Soon I discovered the bathrobe I got for 20 per cent off went down another 10 per cent the following day. I always cut the price tags the moment I got home. A bad habit! I had done the same for the bathrobe and could not bring it to the store to get some money back when the price went down. I was mad at myself. Soon the prices of these goods were cut by 40 per cent, then by 50 per cent, and it was not even Christmas. I wondered if prices might go down to a third of what was originally listed when the holiday drew closer and perhaps would be marked down to a quarter of its value in the new year. I was not around to find out.

I did not know that I was such an avaricious consumer and to be kinder to myself, a shopper with a strong acquisitive instinct. I did not go for the expensive items and what I bought was on sale; still, the numbers would add up. New purchases began piling up, taking up the already limited space in our downsized retirement home. Two weeks into the mall exercise I told myself I had to be disciplined and stop buying things I did not need. I could follow the two women's example to turn around at the store entrance, but I was too weak to resist the temptation of the displays. I walked in believing I could be strong like the two men I saw every day, to focus on the path ahead and ignore the two sides. This was wishful thinking.

I was a little better in the next two weeks than in the first two, but I was not always successful in stopping myself from looking or buying. I was easily distracted or attracted by the sale signs, especially when the price went way down. I would wander off the path, forage the goods, and sometimes make the detour to the cashier. When I was paying for a shirt sold at half the original price, I confessed to the assistant that I was supposed to be exercising not buying things. By that time, perhaps, even the sales personnel recognized me with my almost daily visits; she smiled and said, "This is shopping aerobics."

"Shopping aerobics" was the most interesting and exhilarating activity in those early weeks of radiation, perhaps since receiving my diagnosis of breast cancer, and remained that way for a long time after the active treatment phase. Walking the mall might have seemed mundane and even boring before cancer treatment; now I found it interesting, offering me just the right kind of exercise for my level of energy. It was a much-relished, exciting distraction from the routine of radiation or the boredom of staying home. I could not tell the physical benefits of the workout on my legs, but I could certainly appreciate the psychological one. For half an hour or more each day, I forgot my troubles. My mind was completely taken off cancer, off treatment, and off any physical or emotional discomforts. I scoured the stores for sales, bought what I fancied, and felt normal like the other customers walking and shopping in the mall. It was a true diversion. No wonder the medical profession recommends those suffering from chronic illness to engage in enjoyable activities to take their minds off the ordeal. They suggest taking up painting, reading, playing music, sewing, crochet, walking, or other such hobbies; I have not come across shopping. I bet no one has ever thought of it! My diversion was shopping. It made me feel good and upbeat. I was even following medical advice!

My shopping spree might have been a little costly and the purchase wasteful, but this form of diversion that gave me an emotional uplift was a real bargain when compared to what I would have to pay if I had sought professional help for the same purpose. A brief visit to a counselor or a psychologist would cost me much more; to see one five days a week would add up to a fortune, and these visits might not have produced the same positive results as my shopping aerobics. My kind of diversion worked. The colorful displays lifted my spirit; looking at them was visual pleasure, and touching them was sheer sensual delight. Discovering an item that I liked was exciting, to find one that fit was exhilarating, and taking possession of one at a good price got my adrenaline pumping. And for sure I would not have anything tangible to show talking to a therapist; my trophies from the stores are safe at the back of the closet, and I can take them out to admire or show them off once in a while. In retrospect, perhaps spending money on these items of little use was not wasteful after all; it was money well spent.

The morning radiation together with shopping aerobics wiped me out completely for the rest of the day. Once home, I would grab whatever was available to eat. These were usually the pork shank house specials left in the slow cooker or in the fridge to be heated in the microwave. Then it was nap time. I would fall asleep to wake up a little before five. Dinner was a medley of meat, vegetables, or other ingredients I had dumped in the slow cooker earlier in the afternoon, or it might have been the same food I had for lunch. Either way, I filled my stomach. It was no later than eight in the evening before I was back in bed again for the night's sleep – a much-needed rest to get me ready for another day of radiation, arm exercise, and shopping aerobics.

ELEVEN

Weekend of Anguish

The brochure from Grace Hospital recommended daily arm exercise; this was nothing more than stretching the arm in different directions to break the scarred tissue built up during healing, loosen the muscles, and restore the range of arm movement that could have been compromised as a result of the breast cancer operation. It was also to forestall lymphedema, commonly known as elephant arm – fluid retention that sometimes occurs in the upper arm when a large number of lymph nodes are removed. I did not have lymphedema, but I suffered from shoulder pain and restricted arm movement. I did the arm exercises with effort and in pain, but I noticed my range of arm movement improving. I continued the exercise routine and did not stop when I was receiving radiation.

Five weeks into radiation I was doing arm stretches as I had been doing every evening before going to bed, when I noticed something wet on the front of my pajamas.

"Stupid! Splashing water brushing teeth!" I scolded myself; a habit of talking to myself had developed when I lived alone as a student.

A little while after I got into bed, the sheet over me was wet. The liquid could not have come from careless tooth-brushing; it had to come from somewhere else, and most likely from inside me. Something was wrong. I did not know what it was. I was worried. Victor was sound asleep, tired from all the extra responsibilities loaded on him during the day; I did not wake him up. In any case, there was nothing much he could do at this time on a Friday night.

The next morning, I put on a clean top and soon found two wet spots where the surgeon had taken out the tumor; I put on another top, and it got wet in the same two locations. I inspected the incision in the mirror but could find nothing unusual, and neither could Victor. The fluid had to have seeped out from pin-sized holes too small for the naked eye to see, and whatever it was appeared to be color- and odorless. I did not know what to make of it or what to do.

Victor is never short of ideas and always quick to make suggestions, and many of them. Since my cancer diagnosis, he had not been his usual self. He was unusually quiet and did not say much. He did not fight back even when I snapped at him for no good reason. In the past he would counter any verbal attacks with sharp retorts, especially if they were uncalled for or unprovoked, and sometimes he might be the aggressor initiating these offensives. In the last two months I was the aggressive one and he the silent victim. When decisions had to be made, he stayed on the sidelines while I called the shots doing things my way. He would only offer comments when I asked for his opinion, and he would extend a restraining hand ever so gently when he felt I was heading too far in a very wrong direction. This display of passivity and consideration was a side of him I had not seen before. That Saturday he kept this up and did not make any comments or give any advice on the leaking incision.

Radiation inflamed and reddened my skin, but the procedure did not give me blisters as it does to some recipients with lighter skin. The leaking incision did not hurt and the fluid was clear. Instinct told me something like this should not happen and was something I should not ignore; I had to see a doctor. However, I would not be able to reach one on a weekend, and I did not feel the situation was so urgent that I had to go to the emergency room either. If I did, it would be a long, uncomfortable wait of three to four hours, maybe longer, in a crowded room, and more than likely the doctor on duty would send me home to see my own physician without doing anything. I knew the problem, whatever it might be, would not kill me, at least not at the moment; I would wait until Monday. My lack of urgency, however, did not mean that I did not worry.

Just as the day when I was diagnosed with cancer, I turned to my readily accessible web doctor and revisited the sites I had consulted earlier. I used search words like wound healing, wound opening, incision opening, incision closing, radiation, and any other relevant terms I could think of to shed light on the problem and found no information on an opened incision that was once closed. The websites mentioned color changes, burned skin, blisters, fatigue, pain, rib damage, lung damage, heart damage, and other fallouts from radiation on the breast but made no reference to fluid oozing from the wound. I scoured the blogs, forums, and chat rooms of breast cancer patients; the participants talked about fatigue, burned skin, blisters, and other reactions but again made no mention of leakages.

I never really got an answer to what was happening; even when I saw Dr. McEwan the following week, she did not explain to me why the incision leaked. In her final treatment report, however, she attributed it to seroma developed during radiation; I got a copy of the document from the radiation clinic when my treatment was over. Getting the medical records from the three doctors after the active treatment phase was a precautionary measure; no one knew what lay ahead. The information in this most recent round of treatment may be a useful reference for the next medical team if and when cancer should come back.

According to the web doctor, seroma is the accumulation of fluid at a surgical site that sometimes occurs after an operation, which is why surgeons oftentimes secure a tube at the incision for drainage. However, this might not be needed in minor surgery, and I did not get one when my tumor was taken out. To attribute the leaking to the presence of seroma does not provide the full answer, though. Dr. McEwan identified the source of the fluid but not why it came out in the middle of radiation. Moreover, seroma did not develop during radiation as she had claimed. The stretched skin on my breast after surgery was a telltale sign of fluid inside; I knew my breast and knew it was swollen, but I thought it was normal for the breast to look like this after an operation. I did not think much about it since it did not hurt. I trusted the doctors would see the swelling when they examined my breast and would do something about it if it was a problem. Apparently both the surgeon and the radiation oncologist missed it.

The incision closed with the fluid still inside, and perhaps zapping the breast with X-rays (and I hope not a miscalculated overly strong dosage) weakened the two spots to release it. This is my interpretation of what happened. No one, not even the doctor looking after me at the time, had bothered to find out and I never got the answer. The lack of interest in finding out what was going on and how or why it happened when it happened upset me a lot. It seemed no one cared, and I could not help feeling abandoned. No one could imagine my anguish at the time.

That weekend I searched for answers and found none. When I was first diagnosed with breast cancer, I got information on the web and felt reassured. Now I got no information on the internet and no assurance; I was not even aware that seroma could be a possible explanation. I was completely in the dark and felt totally lost. With no answers, I could only ask questions. What was happening to my body? Where did this liquid come from? Why did the incision leak? Finding no information, I could only speculate and conjured up the worst. Since the incision opened while I was receiving radiation, the procedure had to be the trigger. Radiation should not have opened the incision once it closed, but it did. Could it be too much radiation? Did the medical physicist or the dosimetrist make a mistake in the calculations? Was the X-ray too strong? The number of radiation sessions had been raised, was it too many? What would be the fallout? I had read about the many damages radiation could do to the body. High dosage of radiation is carcinogenic. If this was the case, exposures to overly strong X-rays that opened the incision once healed could do harm. There would be serious consequences waiting for me; the possibilities frightened me.

In a split second, the stoic took over. I had to face the challenge. If a mistake had been made during radiation, what had been done was done; I could not turn back the clock. The questions then changed – What did I have to do to stop the leaking? What could I do to limit the damage? Should I stop radiation for now? For good? And I could not help asking, what would come of the opened incision? Would it open completely? If it did, then what? Again, the lack of answers tortured me. These questions surfaced again and again over the weekend and in the days to follow.

I might have appeared sedate and composed, like the day when I first learned of my breast cancer, but I was not the same. I was no longer the same self-assured woman who searched for information, found the answers, called the doctors, and arranged for treatment. Cancer is not a disease where the person sees a doctor, gets a prescription, takes the medicine, and is good in no time. Getting cancer and receiving treatment is a drawn-out process more like living through an earthquake. After the initial shock, one is sure more shocks will come, but no one can predict how many more or how and when the natural disaster will run its course. One is never sure if the quake just experienced is part of the foreshock and wonders when the main shock and aftershock will follow. The same goes for anyone living through cancer. The diagnosis of cancer is only the opening salvo, more tests will follow, and then there is treatment. Surgery, radiation, and chemotherapy follow the initial diagnosis in a cancer earthquake; these procedures are devastating and draining, and more so if they bring unwanted side effects. Surgery and radiation to rid me of the malignant cancer cells had brought physical discomfort; the procedures had also weakened my soul, eroding my emotional fortitude and verve. I was nervous, anxious, and fearful.

The leaking wound was the last straw to break this camel's back in the drawn-out process of getting "cured." It did not give me additional physical suffering, but I agonized over not knowing what was happening to my body, why it was happening, what it did to my body, and what I had to do about it. The initial shock and the physical and emotional discomforts of treatment were nothing compared to what I was experiencing. The uncertainty that came from not knowing what was going on was mental and emotional torture with a much higher reading on the Richter scale of cancer shocks than any of the earlier ones. The tectonic plates were shifting under my feet and the ground was opening up; I was about to fall in and be swallowed by the earth.

I had to find help. None of my medical friends specialized in oncology; they would still know more than me and might throw light on the subject. I called a geriatrician friend; she did not have the answer and offered to consult a colleague in the field. In the meantime, I called other medical friends. For the first time I learned how cautious medical professionals could be; none would venture a diagnosis or provide a recommendation without seeing the patient. I got no explanation or suggestions; my geriatrician friend kept her word and emailed what her radiation oncologist friend told her – the earlier radiation sessions target the whole breast and the boost, the last few sessions, focus on the tissues around the tumor where vagrant cancer cells are most likely to be found. This was generic information, not exactly what I was looking for, but it was the closest answer I could get.

I could understand why doctors would not make a recommendation sight unseen, but their caution was of no help to me. Only when treatment was over did these professionals feel comfortable giving me a straight answer; every single one said I should have stopped radiation. When I visited Hong Kong with the treatment behind me, a high school friend practicing family medicine compared my situation to patients undergoing chemotherapy. Doctors delay or stop chemotherapy when patients have low white blood cell counts; I should have held off radiation at least until the leaking stopped and the incision healed. Her opinion was seconded by a retired radiation oncologist I met recently. When I told him my story, he was direct.

"We wait for the incision to close before starting radiation; the doctor should have done the same – stop radiation to let the wound heal."

What the two doctors said made sense. I wish someone had said that to me at the time.

Since I could not get an answer from medical friends, I turned to friends who had had radiation for breast cancer treatment. The result was the same; I did not get the information or advice but for a different reason – they had not had this problem and had never heard of it. Misery seeks company. The uniqueness of my problem did not make me feel special; it only increased my sense of isolation and despair.

A friend, if I should even call her one, responded to my query in an email: "You pushed it."

She might as well have said, "You asked for it." Kicking a drowning dog! Blaming the victim! No different from holding women responsible for bringing rape onto themselves! It was the clothes they wore or did not wear and the way they carried themselves. I had told this person I wanted to see Father as soon as possible, but the desire to see him did not translate into pressuring a doctor to do something I was not ready for. I was not so stupid as to do that, and no doctor in her right mind would let a patient push her to do something that might bring such dire consequences. And how did she know I pushed the doctor to give me radiation before I was ready in the first place? I did not do such a thing and never told her I did. She jumped to conclusions without looking at the facts and judged me unfairly. It was bad enough to suffer through the uncertainties and not know what was happening or what to do about it and to be blamed for bringing a medical complication that was so troubling and of which I had no control! It hurt. She had just added another notch on my Richter scale of cancer shocks.

I was livid. I cannot imagine what I would have done if she had said it to my face. I could have yelled at her even though it was not in my nature to do so. In my fury, I emailed three words in response – "I did not" – and never heard from her again.

I told Victor about the exchange. He said my friend did not mean it that way, but I could see no other way to read her statement and refused to be consoled.

It was late Sunday afternoon, more than forty hours since the leaking started, and it had not stopped. I was exhausted with all the questions running through my mind and no closer to an explanation or solution; I had to know what to do and where to go for help on Monday. I had to ask medical friends for suggestions. I called Stephen who was in family practice. When he picked up the phone, I told my story and was careful to explain that I was not looking for a diagnosis or treatment recommendation, I only wanted to know where and how to get medical help. He was diplomatic and said if he were in my shoes, he would call the surgeon and the radiation oncologist. I was relieved to have a game plan.

Again, my desire for a dream team surfaced. I had been seeing three doctors, each operating independently and not communicating with one another. If I had a team of specialists working together, I might not be in this bind. There would be a team leader or a front person for me to contact and perhaps by this time I would know the person well enough to feel comfortable enough to call on a weekend. I would be spared of the weekend of anguish.

TWELVE

Lost

I called Dr. McEwan, the radiation oncologist, and Dr. Shield, the surgeon, first thing Monday morning to resolve my medical problem. It was not exactly eight o'clock, but it was close; I knew the offices might not be open, but I could not wait. Even if they were open, the staff might not answer the phone and I might have to talk to a machine. I might dislike talking to a machine, but it could be useful; I could count on it to get my message through. I was not to be disappointed. The machines were turned on, so I explained my problem and asked for an appointment to see the doctor.

I seemed to wait for ages, but Dr. Shield's nurse returned the call not long after I left the message.

"Do you have pus coming out from the wound?" she asked.

"I don't know. I have fluid coming out of the incision."

I was not exactly sure what pus from an incision would look like. She sensed my ignorance and probed me with more questions.

"Is it thick?"

"No," I replied.

"Is it green?"

"No," I repeated.

"Does it smell?"

"No," I answered in the negative for a third time.

"Dr. Shield will see you if Dr. McEwan sends you."

I was so pleased when Dr. Shield told me at our first meeting that I could call him any time I needed help; it turned out to be an empty offer. Yes, I could call him any time but reaching him was another question. I had to get past his gatekeeper but I could not. Like the employee in Dr. Gray's office, Dr. Shield's nurse would not let me through. She did not exactly turn me down, but she imposed a pre-requisite – I had to get another doctor's referral; it was a no just the same. If I could see Dr. McEwan, I might not need the surgeon. I did not say this to her, though; I only said it in my head.

When a friend heard what happened, she told me with a smile, if not a smirk, that I would have gotten the attention if I had answered in the affirmative to all three questions. Hindsight is always twenty-twenty. I stayed away from the doctors too much and for too long to know how things worked, and I did not have the skills to ask the right questions or give the correct response. I gave the wrong answers. It was not the first or last time I made such mistakes. My ineptness in navigating the system ruined my chance to get the medical help I so desperately needed. I suffered the consequences and paid the hefty price. Like the medical doctors who told me that I was to have stopped radiation when the incision opened, this friend's advice came a little too late.

Dr. McEwan called almost the moment I put down the phone talking with Dr. Shield's nurse. I explained my problem to the doctor, and she asked me to come in fifteen minutes before the usual radiation time. After a weekend of anguish, a doctor would finally look at my breast! Help was on the way, and to be more accurate I was on my way to get help. I could breathe again!

"Thank you," I said with gratitude emanating from the bottom of my heart.

I had been wearing tops with a couple of buttons open, easy to put on and take off in those days of radiation. I put on a clean one and the stained one went into a bag.

"Just like Monica Lewinsky's dress."

The blue semen-stained dress the White House intern Lewinsky turned over to the special counsel prosecutor investigating President Bill Clinton in 1998 got the latter into trouble; mine would get me out of it. The stained top would help the doctor diagnose the problem and decide what to do. I smiled at the comparison not knowing it would be a long, long time before I would smile again.

It was past eight o'clock, so we had to hurry to make the appointment at nine fifteen. We were in the car in no time with Victor behind the wheel and his foot on the gas pedal, perhaps pressing a little too hard. Speeding the whole way, we were at the radiation clinic only a few minutes late.

Dr. McEwan was in her usual attire, a white coat over her light-colored blouse, dark pants, and dark loafers, seemingly the standard work clothes of the medical practitioners in my cancer care. Her flaming red hair that usually cascaded down her shoulders was pulled back into a knot, giving her a severe look. She did not give me her hallmark smile when she walked into the room, but her solemn countenance did not alarm me; a doctor would be concerned if her patient had a problem.

I repeated what I told her over the phone.

"I found the stains Friday evening ... wetting the blanket.... It leaked the whole weekend.... Leaking has not stopped."

To emphasize what I said, I took the neatly folded T-shirt from the bag, flapped it open, and held it up with the stains facing the doctor. She took one look at it from six feet away and showed no interest in examining it further.

I was a little annoyed at the lack of interest in my exhibit and unbuttoned my top. She took the cue, got up from her chair, and walked over to where I was sitting with my bare breast. She bent down to look. Victor and I could not locate the openings over the weekend; it would be difficult for her to find them if I were lying down on the examination table, and it would be almost impossible for her to see anything while standing over me. That was why I brought the top.

After a brief look, with her hands at her side and never touching my breast, she straightened up and walked back to her chair. She looked straight at me and said slowly in a low but audible voice.

"It's all right. We can continue radiation."

I came to her with high hopes; what I got was a disappointment. She had not really looked at the T-shirt; she had not really examined the wound. She took a split-second look at my breast and made the decision to do nothing as if nothing had happened. Perhaps I should not say that; she was doing something – she was continuing radiation, inaction disguised as action. Alright to continue radiation? And only that? I had no idea what the doctor would do when I came to see her; but I did not expect this.

I had not compared my situation to patients having low white blood cell counts during chemotherapy, nor had I thought of patients waiting for the incision to close after surgery before starting radiation. In some vague way, however, I had perhaps associated radiation with the leaking wound, considered it the culprit, and in my subconscious I had probably wanted to halt the procedure temporarily if not for good.

I did not have any plan of action on my way to see the doctor. I had no intention of doing what I was about to do and had to have been very upset with her decision in order to do it. My next move said it all. I was not about to let go.

I had been perplexed when Dr. Gray's nurse gave me the three doctors' phone numbers, but I had not asked her to explain. I had not asked Dr. Shield to elaborate on the pros and cons of lumpectomies and mastectomies when I knew the information was essential for me to make a choice between the two. And I had not asked the radiation oncologist to explain when I was curious about the increase in the number of radiation sessions from twenty to thirty-three. It was simply not in my nature to ask questions in medical offices; I remained quiet even when I should have spoken up. And I was about to contradict the doctor's decision – a big departure from my usual hesitance to open my mouth in a doctor's office!

I read over the weekend on the American Cancer Society website that women over seventy with stage 1 hormone-positive breast cancer may not need to have radiation after surgery if the tumors are small; this was the type of breast cancer I had. I did not know the exact reason behind the recommendation. I only knew that studies had shown that the additional treatment did not do much to lower the chances of the cancer returning. By that time, I had read enough to realize that medical treatment is a balancing game. There are always risks involved with any medical intervention, and the benefits of the treatment have to be weighed against the possible harmful side effects, with the balance between the two varying from situation to situation and from patient to patient. This recommendation is probably based on weighing the slow growth of cancer cells at this age and the undesirable side effects of radiation. I was not seventy, but I was getting close with only three years to go. In any event, cutoff points are somewhat arbitrary. Why seventy? What if the woman is sixty-nine?

"Women over seventy do not need radiation. The American Cancer Society said so," I said softly.

I did not say it straight out, but the message was clear. I was telling the doctor I did not agree with her decision; I wanted radiation to stop temporarily, if not for good. I was "pushing" the oncologist, as my friend had intimated earlier when she blamed me for pressuring the doctor to give me the radiation. I quoted the cancer society's recommendation and leaned on an authority. I had never before argued with a doctor let alone challenged one; I did just that.

If Dr. McEwan was listening, she did not hear what I said. If she had heard my words, she might not have understood. If she had understood, the message did not register. If she had gotten the message, she did not agree with me. And she ignored me! She and I might as well have been speaking different languages.

The doctor looked at me with the same solemn expression she had when she walked into the room and when she told me radiation had to continue.

"Radiation kills cancer cells. It's important to do that." She said slowly and quietly.

She said nothing new. She just repeated a truism that should be reconsidered under the circumstances. She might not be using the same words in her earlier message, but the message was the same – radiation had to continue. And she said it in a serious and studied manner, a complete turn-around from her usual flamboyant friendliness! Gone was the pleasant and gregarious doctor who shared with me her social and family life! She had become the distant, stern medical practitioner issuing a directive to her patient.

Radiation kills cancer cells. I knew that! That's why I came to her in the first place! That was the reason for radiation. Medicine is a science and an art; treatment has to be adapted to the circumstances and to the patient's situation. That was what the American Cancer Society was saying when it recommended radiation for younger patients but not so much for older ones. In my case, the situation had changed; the incision was leaking. Was I to disregard the opened incision? What if the incision opened further with more radiation? Those were my thoughts, but I did not articulate them. I became once again the quiet patient reticent to voice her opinion.

I told her what I wanted. My preference was clear, and she ignored it. I leaned on the authority of the American Cancer Society to ask her to reconsider her decision, but it did not work. I had nothing to add. I did not know the subject, and I could not think of any other reason to back me up. The social scientist in me would not allow me to take a position unless it was supported by evidence. I did not know much about breast cancer and knew even less about radiation. If I knew why the incision opened, I might know how to stop it. I might be able to argue my case. I did not. I only wanted to stop radiation. This was how I felt; it was not an informed position. How could I defend what I would like to do? How could I justify it? I could give no evidence or reason.

Some have suggested that patients should be their own advocates; I tried and had failed. I was not up to the task. I did not agree with the doctor and did not like where she was taking me; I feared the consequences of continued radiation, but I did not know how to bring her over to my side. My instincts told me something was wrong, but what exactly that was I did not know. Instinct also told me continuing radiation could do more harm than good, though I did not know why. All I had were gut feelings. How could I defend instinct and gut feelings? To continue arguing by repeating the American Cancer Society's recommendation would look silly and give the impression that I was trying to pick a fight with the doctor. I knew it would be of no use to say anything more, because she would not change her mind. I was back to my normal behavior in medical offices and kept my thoughts to myself. I remained silent.

I could have walked away from this doctor. I had read in more than one article that some patients who are unhappy with their doctors look for others. I did not know how to find other doctors and was too cautious to try. Where would I find another radiation oncologist? I could ask Dr. Gray, but doctors sometimes recommend their friends in their referrals; Dr. McEwan might be a friend. If this was the case, how could I tell him I wanted to drop his friend halfway through radiation and ask him to recommend another? In any case, I might not get past Dr. Gray's gatekeepers; they might shut me out again. I could rely on word of mouth to find one. I had a few friends who received radiation for breast cancer treatment, but none lived in town; they would not know any radiation oncologists here. I could turn to the internet; common sense told me I could not always trust everything on the web when accolades could be manufactured or simply paid self-advertisements. Even if I had a pool of doctors to choose from, what criteria should I use to pick the person? What qualities would I be looking for? If I did go down that path, there was no guarantee the second would be any better than the first. It was a risk I could not and did not want to take. It would take time and energy I did not have to do the search, so I never seriously considered this alternative.

I have considered myself a rebel, rejecting the shibboleth to obey those higher in the social hierarchy. My Chinese upbringing told me to do what the elders said; growing up I had time and time again defied my parents to do the exact opposite of what I was told. I resented the practice of bowing to higher-ups in the bureaucracy and had stood up to the university administration, telling them I disagreed and sometimes telling them they were wrong only to earn their displeasure. As for deferring to the rich, whoever wanted me to do so could simply forget this and save their energy trying. I have always followed logic and trusted experts. Knowledge is power; the knowledgeable makes informed decisions and takes judicious action. I buy into this, and when translated into action, it gives those with knowledge authority and suggests acquiescence from those without. Dr. McEwan was the expert in radiation oncology and was supposed to know; I was the ignorant patient who did not know any better, which was why I was in her office. Even though I disagreed with her decision I could not shake off my decades of social science training and practice.

I cannot help thinking of Talcott Parsons, the conservative sociology guru, when I write these pages. He argued that doctors, with their training and expertise, were the ones to bring patients back to health; therefore they occupied an authoritative if not authoritarian position in the doctor-patient relationship. Liberal social scientists like Paul Starr, however, criticized Parsons's exclusive focus on the physicians' expertise in this dyadic relationship. They went beyond his narrow focus to point to the social, political, and economic factors contributing to the physicians' inordinate social status and how the profession had managed to create and maintain their superior position over time. I have never bought into Parsons's analysis either, because I can see how his arguments can be used to justify the status quo and to ignore the inequities and problems in existing social arrangements.

It is ironic that despite my reservations with Parsons's analysis, my deliberations followed exactly his line of thinking, and I acted exactly as he would have predicted or expected a patient to. The doctor's wishes prevailed; I made the decision to do what Dr. McEwan told me because of our asymmetry in medical knowledge – she knew better what to do. And it is more ironic or sad to say that my preference, not hers, turned out to overlap with what other disinterested medical personnel would have recommended. My decision to trust her expert knowledge turned out to be misplaced.

This doctor might not see herself as a god, but she became my goddess of medicine just the same. I put my reservations aside, relinquished independent thinking, suspended judgment, put my faith in her, and believed that my trust was well placed. I joined ranks with my many fellow cancer patients who followed their doctors' direction without question. Their mantra on the cancer journey became mine – "In doctors we trust." In my obeisance to this doctor, Tennyson's "The Charge of the Light Brigade" came to mind:

Theirs not to make reply
Theirs not to reason why
Theirs but to do and die.

I could only hope the last line would read:

Theirs but to do and survive.

There were times I wondered why patients trusted Farid Fata, the oncologist found guilty of millions of dollars of medical fraud with some patients receiving chemotherapy when they had no cancer. Now I understand. For whatever and different reasons, patients trust the experts, believe in them, and do what they say. When a doctor tells someone he or she is sick, the person becomes a patient. When the doctor offers chemotherapy or any treatment procedure, the patient welcomes it as a remedy. It is hard to break away from the trust we put in medical practitioners. I have considered myself an independent thinker and skeptical of the aura, perks, and privileges doctors enjoy, yet I accepted Dr. Gray's statement that I had cancer when I did not feel anything different and underwent surgery. Now that I had doubts and every fiber of my being revolted against Dr. McEwan's decision, I still could not tear myself away from this trust in doctors; I did not feel confident enough to break away to do something different or have the audacity to defy her. I submitted to her wishes and followed her directive.

This was a cataclysmic fall for this Chinese woman professor who broke glass ceilings, stood confidently in front of one cohort of university students after another, and argued with the university administration to become this compliant, feckless patient. My former male colleagues would not have believed this was the same woman who had tangled with and stood up to them. My obeisance to the doctor was a far cry from the headstrong female professional who took matters into her own hands over the years or the belligerent patient who charted her own treatment course only two months earlier.

I exchanged my street clothes for the patient gown – the cotton swathe cloth with only strings to secure it over my naked body – the attire of subordinates in the temple of the medical goddess signaling ultimate submission and subservience. The analogy might be unfair, but this was how I felt. I bowed my head and dragged my feet on the seemingly endless trek to the radiation bunker. After all, I was not the brave soldier of Tennyson's Light Brigade charging fearlessly into the Valley of Death at the leader's command. I was the cowardly, reluctant recruit who did not see eye to eye with her commander and was too weak to stand her ground. When my commander pointed out the direction, I did not march; I dragged my feet and slowly plodded down the path, hoping it would not lead into my Valley of Death when I had already passed the jaws of "living" hell.

I climbed slowly onto the radiation table and stayed limp while Ruby and John performed the usual pushing and pulling routine. When they were done, they left the room with me lying perfectly still on the table – the sacrificial lamb on the altar waiting for the X-ray lightning to strike. I no longer counted my numerals in Cantonese; I did not need to. My mind was preoccupied, racing with questions.

"Therapeutic nihilism?"

"Radiation to be pursued at any cost?"

"What would happen to the leakage in the wound?"

"What if the wound opens up?"

These new questions and others that tortured me over the weekend kept surfacing and resurfacing, circling in my head. I told myself to stop asking these questions; doing that would do me no good and only add to my aggravation. I tried to stop thinking, but I could not; my brain was running at full speed, raising questions that had no answers.

A true healer does not cure the disease and ignore the patient. What is the point of "healing" when the patient does not want the remedy, feels miserable with what is prescribed, or simply does not want to be healed? When the medical professional organizations remind doctors to be patient-centered they seem to be stating the obvious; after all, what is medical care without the patient? What is the purpose of medicine if it is not to benefit the patient? These professional organizations are probably aware of these possible anomalous situations when patients do not want the particular treatment for one reason or another to remind doctors to be patient-centered, to respect patients, and to take patient wishes into consideration when deciding what to do. In my case the doctor was so preoccupied with clinical concerns she ignored the patient. Killing cancer cells seemed to be Dr. McEwan's paramount concern; she forgot that the body that housed these cancer cells was a human person. She did not seem to care what this person thought or felt, let alone to take the person's preferences into consideration in her decision-making.

I did not know about patient-centeredness at the time. I resented Dr. McEwan's clinical preoccupation and rankled at her arrogance to stick to her decision to continue radiation. She brushed aside what I told her, did not investigate the problem, and ignored the changed circumstances. She was so self-assured with what she was doing. If she had looked at the stains on my clothes, examined the incision, or explained the reasoning behind her action, I might have felt better about her decision even if I had reservations. She did not do any of the above. She did not have enough respect for this patient to listen to or try to understand where I was coming from. I was nothing; what I said did not count and was not worth considering. She did not see the patient and human person before her. I might have a radiation oncologist "looking after" me, but I felt abandoned just the same.

Perhaps my submission to her directive upset me more and made me feel worse. I have always enjoyed reading books on the French Revolution and other insurrections. I admired the Ho Chi Minhs and Che Guevaras of the world and found these revolutionaries courageous, their exploits exciting, sometimes even seeing myself as one of them. My behavior in the radiation clinic, however, revealed that I was not a rebel; I was a coward not worthy to be counted among the revolutionary ranks. The downtrodden recognized the flaws in the system and knew what had to be changed; some knew how to change it, and others had the courage to act on it. I did not have the perspicuity to understand what was going on, the knowhow to identify a solution, or the courage to change the situation. I was ignorant of the disease, the treatment procedures, the workings of the medical system, or what could be done to resolve the problem. I had no overseer watching my back, no chains on my legs, no four walls closing in around me, yet I felt compelled to do what I was told. I resented the doctor telling me to continue radiation. I did not agree with the path chosen, but I did not have the courage to say no or do anything otherwise, so I submitted to something I did not want. The revelations hurt.

THIRTEEN

Days of Hell

I met with Dr. McEwan each Wednesday after the treatment session. At these meetings the doctor would ask how I felt, and I would report that my skin was red and I was tired but otherwise nothing unusual; she took me at my word and never examined my breast. I did not like stripping in front of a doctor, man or woman; not having to do that was fine with me. The encounter would be over in a minute without our social exchanges. After a couple of weeks, I knew all about her kids, the schools they attended, the sports they played, her weekend golf, and their holidays in Florida. I am a private person and rarely reciprocated the information. Even with these add-ons, the meeting would be over in five minutes.

Two days after I "resumed" radiation I had the usual Wednesday consultation with the doctor. Dr. McEwan was back to her cheery self, big smile, and sprightly gait. She asked the usual questions, but she did not get the usual answers; I told her the wound was still leaking. There was an examination table in the room, but she did not ask me to lie down for her to take a look.

I was worried about the leaking and what would come of the incision with the continued radiation. Before she could begin her usual social chat, I asked, "What will happen if the incision opens further?" This had been on my mind when the leaking started over the weekend and more so with continued radiation without anything being done to the opened wound; I didn't get anything to help the healing. Fluid had continued to escape from invisible holes and the problem could get worse; the incision opening was a real possibility. The question was valid, but I had something more in mind. It was my roundabout way to ask her to reconsider the decision, another plea to her to stop radiating me, and another indication of my subconscious determination to stop radiation.

The diplomacy did not work; the doctor did not catch the subtext in my question, or if she did she ignored it. She took my query literally and answered in her usual lighthearted way.

"The surgeon will open it and close it again."

My eyes opened wide. I could not believe my ears. Just that – open and close the incision again! She accepted the incision opening a possibility, but it didn't seem to matter. It's not a problem. If that happened the surgeon would open and close it. Just like that? So casual!

I might have stayed away from doctors as much as possible all these years, but I respect and trust these trained professionals to have the patient's interest at heart, to cure, to heal, to make patients well again, and I go to them when I have an illness that will not go away. I trust they will cure and heal; this is my expectation of doctors. I had trusted this radiation oncologist, took her suggestion for radiation treatment, and continued the procedure as she told me to do when I had reservations doing that. I believed she knew better and trusted her judgment; I believed she had the patient's interest in mind, and I did what I was told.

I might not have known as much as I do now about when I should commit to radiation and if under the present circumstances I should be getting the treatment at all, but even then her cavalier attitude and remark upset me and made me question if she was a true healer. The leakage was not a problem; she admitted that continued radiation might open the incision, but again it was not a problem. What would constitute a problem? She recognized continued radiation might not allow the incision a chance to close, yet she stayed on course, giving the patient the maximum number of radiation sessions a breast cancer patient could take. What did she have in mind? Was it her overconfidence that prompted her to stick with her original decision? Or was it stubbornness and inflexibility? I did not know. It seemed her priority was to kill the cancer cells; nothing else mattered, certainly not this patient's wishes or perhaps even her health.

If she was a healer, she was an unfeeling one. In her work as a medical doctor, she might have seen this happening many times and sometimes a lot worse. The opened incision might be something mundane in her experience, nothing to worry about. I knew I would not die from it, but that did not mean I was not worried. She was giving me the facts as to what would be done if the incision was open when radiation was over. In my limited experience as a cancer patient, this was a frightening scenario. To have cancer was bad enough; for the incision to reopen was worse; I never had my breast opened and closed just like that. She had no clue how the patient felt, or maybe she did not care. The happy-go-lucky manner with which she delivered the message offended me. I already felt abandoned when she ignored the opened wound, now I was overwhelmed with anger by her insensitivity. I riled.

Perhaps I should not be surprised; she was the "ultimate" professional. She referred to my breast as "the piece" at our first meeting. "Piece" might be the jargon used among professionals, but it was jarring to my ears; I would like a little show of respect to my body, and I did not like my breast reduced to a "piece." To tell me so casually that the surgeon would open and close the wound again was sheer cruelty. She should have put herself in my shoes; apparently, she did not. If I were in her place, I would be more sympathetic and considerate of the patient's feelings and choose my words more carefully. She could have conveyed the message in a gentler way; she could have shown some empathy or some pretensions of such feelings. A short preamble suggesting that this kind of thing sometimes happened, that medical science could not explain why, and that she was sorry it did happen to me would have made me feel better.

Perhaps some sensitivity training would benefit this doctor. Sensitivity is important in any communication, especially if the doctor wants to know where the patient is coming from, to understand the patient's needs, and to pick the best treatment. Demonstrating sensitivity helps to establish rapport with the patient and put the patient at ease. Doing that gains the patient's trust and gets the person to open up to the doctor; it also makes the patient willing and ready to cooperate with medical directives. Indeed, being sensitive when interacting with patients is essential in implementing patient-centeredness – to understand the patient and to fathom the patient's wishes.

Dr. McEwan reminded me of Dr. H-O-D-A-D, the surgeon in Dr. M. Makary's book *Unaccountable: What Hospitals Won't Tell You and How Transparency Can Revolutionize Healthcare*. The surgeon carried out unnecessary procedures and made mistakes recognized by his colleagues but not the patients; the latter were taken in by his pleasant bedside manner and some remained eternally grateful. It was easy to be taken in by Dr. McEwan; she was pleasant, and other patients had praised her for it. Friendliness is good to break the ice and put patients at ease; however, this is not the only quality to make a good doctor. A doctor needs solid medical knowledge, good medical skills, and a heart for patients' well-being. Dr. McEwan's sociability was winning when everything was going smoothly; when things went wrong, though, she became distant, curt, and unapproachable. She was dismissive and ignored my problem, my wishes, and my feelings. The turnaround in her behavior was a disappointment; it made me feel that her initial friendliness was superficial, inappropriate, and even disingenuous.

I did not fear for my life. Continued radiation would not kill me immediately, though it could bring undesirable fallouts in the future; the detrimental effects from radiation or over-radiation would take time to show. High levels of radiation can increase the risk of getting cancer. If the incision opened with over-radiation, the probability of me getting cancer would go up; and if cancer came back in the future, it would not be a problem for this doctor but for another one. She was not responsible to put things right.

These scenarios were not reassuring. In desperation I called Dr. Gray, even though I had been turned away before and might be rejected again. But I could not think of any other person to turn to. The doctor would know something even though he was not a cancer specialist; he might be able to shed light on what was happening and give me advice. As usual, I reported my problem to the machine and the nurse or receptionist returned my call to tell me one more time the doctor was not looking after my cancer; I had to go to the specialists. Too tired to argue I accepted her answer and hung up.

I had come across many medical websites and literature suggesting that a cancer patient should have an advocate – another pair of ears to listen in case the patient misses or misinterprets what the doctor has said, another mind to help the patient think clearly, and another voice to articulate patient concerns to healthcare providers. This person gives the patient emotional support, holds back rush decisions, and backs her up if she chooses to fight the medical establishment. An informed advocate who knows medicine and is familiar with the workings of the medical system will be all the better to do these tasks. The family doctors who stood by my cancer friends and called the specialists for clarification, explaining to them the report and preparing them for what was to come, was acting in that capacity. This person could not have been more needed, more welcomed, more valued, or more appreciated by me at this time. Perhaps calling Dr. Gray was my last vain attempt to recruit him as one at this late stage of treatment. I failed dismally; I did not even get a chance to talk to him.

When Dr. Gray's gatekeeper rejected me one more time, my sense of being abandoned felt more real and complete. The radiation oncologist stood me up by ignoring my problem, the family doctor did the same by being inaccessible, and my medical friends were distant and noncommittal. I had no medical information, no medical help. I became the rudderless boat in an open sea left at the mercy of the elements with no stars to guide me; the water was black and the cerulean sky dark. It was black all around. I was swallowed by darkness with no idea what had happened, what was happening, what would happen, or how to fend for myself. I did not know what to do or where to turn for help, so I did nothing.

In the days to follow I attended my daily radiation session. It was no longer treatment to get better; it was only an exercise following doctor's orders. Victor drove me to the clinic, waited, and took me home. I stopped walking in Galleria Mall because leg exercise was no longer my priority. I stopped the arm exercises because they might tear the opening further to cause more problems. I stopped examining the opened incision because there was nothing I could see. Even if I saw anything different there was nothing I could do. I stopped answering the phone because there was

nothing I wanted to talk about. I emailed friends to stop calling so I would not be disturbed in my inaction. In my waking hours I rested, which really meant I did not do anything.
I sat in the living room recliner or lay on the bed oblivious
of everything around; I languished. Somnolence was my
daily routine, and I was sad. If anyone wanted to label me
depressed, this would be the time to do it, even though I
still do not think it was depression. Like the time when I
asked Victor how he felt when I was diagnosed with breast
cancer, he said, "You do not expect me to be happy"; with
nothing I could do, you could not expect me to do anything.

On the last day of radiation, Dr. McEwan came into the
treatment room before I could get up from the table and was
her perky self. She was not there to examine the incision; she
had not taken another look at it since the day she declared
it ready for treatment unless one counted the peremptory
glance at my breast the day I came to her with the opened
incision; she came to tell me to make an appointment with
the surgeon and left. My wound needed attention after all!
Now with the radiation sessions over and her part of the
job was done, she gave me the go-ahead to see the surgeon!
Why now? Why not earlier? I could only speculate.

Ruby interrupted my rumination. She had kept an eye on
the opened incision when the doctor ignored it. A couple
of days into my continued radiation she told me she would
ask the doctor to give me something for the wound. She
took the initiative to do something without my asking. Her
pellucid voice never sounded so comforting or soothing
when she told me what she was going to do; she came back
with packages of bacitracin zinc, an antibiotic ointment to

stop infection, probably free samples received from drug companies. She was so different from her employer; she cared for this patient, and her gesture warmed my heart. Someone was keeping an eye on me; her demonstration of concern had probably calmed me and sustained me through those last dark days of radiation. Now she brought me more packages of bacitracin zinc and reminded me to continue applying it on the incision. She was my real ruby, a precious stone dear to my heart then and forever.

At the front office, the receptionist gave me a mug brandishing the logo of the clinic. A souvenir! What cancer patient would want to be reminded of his or her radiation? Not me, especially with my bad experience! They wanted me to come back when cancer returned! The clinic web address and phone number on the mug would tell me where to go. How tacky! The thought revolted me; I wanted to toss it straight into the trash can, but I did not. I did not want to offend the receptionist. She was just the messenger doing what her employer asked her to do, but she might take it personally when I showed such distaste for the "gift" she offered. It would not be fair for me to hurt her feelings. I threw the mug into the garbage the moment I got home.

I was stunned and saddened when I got news of breast cancer and had to delay my trip to see Father in Hong Kong. I accepted the challenges as things that could sometimes happen and needed to be dealt with. To acquire knowledge on cancer and treatment was a steep learning curve; arranging the treatment schedule and waiting to see a doctor was sometimes frustrating; surgery gave me pain and debilities in my shoulder; and radiation drained my energy. Going through all of these was difficult. The incision opening and not finding any answers threw me off; still, I believed that things would be fine once I reached a doctor.

Things did not turn out that way. Instead, I was condemned to a living hell. Dr. McEwan did not see the incision opening as a problem and continued radiation. Her attitude and action signaled her insouciance; reiterating that radiation would kill cancer cells only told me she was stubborn and would not change course. If the treatment procedure was killing the cancer cells inside me, it was also torturing me if not slowly killing me. I was completely lost with nowhere to go and no one to help. I worried about the leaking incision and the fallouts from the "treatment," and I agonized not being able to see Father in Hong Kong. I was miserable.

During this period, I often told myself if the cancer doesn't kill me, the treatment will. I felt normal and did not know the cancerous tumor was in me until I was told. Treatment was supposed to make me better, so I took the bitter medicines. Taking out the tumor and the initial radiation brought physical discomfort, but I trusted the procedures would do me good. Now I had my doubts and questioned what Dr. McEwan was doing. I saw a problem; she did not. She ignored what I saw as a problem and continued radiation. Aside from the physical discomfort from the procedure, I was going through emotional hell. I felt trapped. I did not know how to get out of the quagmire and did not know what to do. I could not get out of the morass and did not know how it would end.

Whenever I thought of the situation, which was often in those last two weeks of radiation, I muttered the same statement to myself: "If cancer doesn't kill me, the treatment will." I might not mean it literally, but it came close. Radiation had continued, and when it was over, the leaking continued and the incision stayed open. I did not know what the damage was and if more was done with the continued radiation. I had no idea what the remedy would be or if there even was one, what medical procedures would follow, and when and how the treatment would end. I worried about the harmful consequences and the cancer waiting around the corner; I did not know when or if I could ever be whole again. Treatment seemed to be a tunnel with no light at the end.

December was the season to be merry, but I was in no mood to celebrate. I was in the doldrums, preoccupied with my troubles, and too tired to take part in any of the festivities going on around me. I could only think of the treatment to follow. My last day of radiation was on December 28; everything in town would come to a standstill, and the medical offices would be closed. I would not be able to see Dr. Gold to get the prescription for adjuvant therapy, and I could not book the appointment to see Dr. Shield to check the open wound. Everything had to wait until the next year. The new year was less than a week away, but under the circumstances the interlude seemed like eons and my days of hell seemed to never come to an end.

FOURTEEN

Grasping for Help

Now that the holidays were over and I could see the surgeon with Dr. McEwan's referral, I should have been elated. But I was restrained and cautious. The last time I rushed to see a doctor for help with optimism and high hopes turned out to be a disappointment; I was miserable and left without hope for too long to dare to raise my expectation lest I would be disappointed again.

The gods of medicine screen all candidates who seek access to their sacred grounds; it was not easy to see the surgeon even with a referral. When I called in the new year, Dr. Shield's gatekeeper gave me an appointment three weeks down the road. After a month of hell, another three weeks with the problem hanging over me and not knowing what was happening or what could happen and not doing anything about it was unacceptable; I impressed on the person answering the call that my problem could not wait. I got an appointment the next week.

The leaking fluid seemed to have dried; the seepage was barely detectable when I examined my clothes; neither did I see anything different when I peeped under the T-shirt. But I could detect a faint putrid odor when I did that. Even my limited medical knowledge told me things were not completely right. Ruby's antibiotic ointment did not work. The wound had not healed, and it might be infected. I had to see a doctor.

Victor had been quiet all this time, but he had to have been very worried because he called Dr. Shield's office after I told him the date of my appointment. He came across strong, as was his normal self; the receptionist could not fend him off and put him through to Michelle the nurse. He got an appointment the very next day. I was not there to hear what he said; I did not even know he made the call. I would not have taken kindly to his intervention behind my back on any other occasion, however well-intentioned. But for once I forgave him, because I wanted an earlier appointment too.

When a friend heard about Victor's success in getting the next-day appointment when I did not, he commented that it was because I am a woman. I am not sure this was the case. True, it does not take a man to discriminate against a woman; women can do the same to their sisters. I experienced put-downs from both men and women inside and outside the workplace time and time again over the years to know that this could happen; in my case such behavior could have been race or gender based. I am sensitive but not hypersensitive with such attitudes and behavior and can usually smell it when it is there. Except for the operator who had difficulty understanding my English when I called for a treatment appointment last September, I did not detect it from anyone else in the three doctors' offices.

The holidays had just ended and the receptionist probably received numerous calls asking to see the surgeon, so I had to wait three weeks. When I pressed for an earlier appointment, she accommodated my request to give me one the next week and I accepted it. Victor felt the urgency to have an even earlier one. He insisted on an earlier date and was rewarded for his insistence and persistence.

I learned a lot about breast cancer, cancer care, and what patients had to deal with on this difficult journey, and I recognized the difficulties their caregivers, family members, and friends had to face. My experience with the three doctors taught me another lesson. When I met Dr. McEwan I was overjoyed to have a woman looking after me. I like to see women taking up prestigious professions once monopolized by men. Besides, I have always believed that women doctors are more sensitive and caring than their male counterparts and give patients closer and better attention. It turned out to not always be the case, at least not for me. This woman doctor's behavior eroded my confidence in the medical profession and the two men restored my faith in it. She ignored the opened incision, but the surgeon stepped in to put things right, and the medical oncologist offered help without my asking. The two men proved to be more sensitive, warmer, and more appreciative of what I had to go through than she did. What happened has warned me to be cautious, avoid stereotyping, and pause before passing judgment in any situation.

What I said here may not go over well with some feminists, and indeed a woman friend who read an earlier draft of the manuscript asked me to use the writer's prerogative to turn the radiation oncologist into a man. Some may see what I described in the preceding pages as tarnishing the reputation of women and undermining what feminists have worked so hard to build; I have no intention to do that. I am not questioning this woman's ability or indeed any woman's ability, nor am I questioning women's caring and nurturing nature in general; I am only saddened by what this doctor did. I do not want to whitewash or deny what happened. I do not want to contribute to the myth of an always good woman or the woman as the perpetual victim. There are good people and bad people, good women and not-so-good ones. Even in the case of sexual harassment, the media has reported cases where the same woman can be victimized by a male higher up in the organization and be a perpetrator taking advantage of a lower-ranking male employee; the unethical exercising power without constraint or restraint is the root of the problem. This doctor did not show concern for my needs and feelings as a good doctor would.

Telling it all does not mean I am any less committed to equity, especially gender equity. I have been a firm believer and ardent supporter of equity since long before the MeToo movement or the Black Lives Matter movement took shape. My own experiences have convinced me that prejudice and discrimination exist and should be eliminated. Prejudice can be based on gender, race, or any other particularistic criteria, and discrimination takes different forms and is expressed in many and often subtle ways. The situation may have improved and might now be better than before. People have become more sensitive to the different kinds of prejudice, and legislation is there to protect minorities from differential treatment. However, loopholes remain and more structural safeguards need to be put in place. Furthermore, values and attitudes are hard to change, and discrimination can sometimes rear its ugly head without the perpetrators recognizing it. Working toward a fair and just society requires vigilance at all times, in all places, with the determined and the joint efforts of both women and men of all races to change the formal and informal social arrangements in the public and private spheres of social life. It will take a long, long time to reach this goal.

Early on the morning of my appointment, Victor and I left the quiet precinct of our residential community to join the vehicles racing along the speedway into town. This town with 300,000 inhabitants had not spawned the concrete jungles of the big cities; the cluster of four- or five-story buildings in the distance marked the town center and did not obscure the outline of the mountains farther away on the distant horizon. Fifteen minutes on the road, the barren expanse we had been driving through gave way to one residential development after another. The houses in each development might have somewhat different elevations to give the illusion they were custom built, but these facades could not hide their origin from the same architectural creator. The transition from one development to the next, however, was stark and very visible. The houses in each had their own unmistakable character; sometimes the community was cordoned off by a brick or concrete rampart, with some separated by an additional aqueduct for rainwater runoff only to remind observers of castle moats. The boxy buildings of groceries, pharmacies, fitness centers, and other retail stores in the commercial plazas completed the suburban landscape.

Soon the single-family homes along the road were replaced by semi-detached ones. These edifices made no pretense to be individualized, with each pair of houses carrying the same outside elevation, the same color walls, and the same tiled roofs, joined in the use of the driveway and separated from its neighbors by the wall they shared. As we got closer to Dr. Shield's office, living arrangements were dense with two-story apartment buildings accommodating four or eight units on each level. Privacy of the unit was guarded by the open space of the parking lots, high windows in the bathrooms, and living room doors to the balcony facing slightly different directions.

This was not what I saw the day I went to see Dr. Shield; it was how I remembered the route I had traveled so many times before. Since the incision started leaking with nothing I could do I retreated into a shell of nothingness doing nothing, oblivious to everything, and barely feeling anything. Victor was the driver in more sense than one, and I allowed myself to be driven. I was no different that day; I was the broken robot on the passenger seat to be delivered to the medical mechanic to be examined and repaired.

Dr. Shield walked into the examination room as his same calm self and in the same blue scrubs with Michelle, the nurse, behind him. The tan I noticed at our first meeting had long faded to give way to his natural copper-tone skin. Four steps past the threshold, he made a sharp left turn to face Victor and me sitting along the wall next to the entrance. We had been bathing in the rays of the warm January sun streaming through the window; now the sun was warming the doctor's back and we were in his shadow.

Unlike the other two doctors Dr. Shield never shook hands with patients; he acknowledged their presence with the opening line, "How can I help you?" He did the same that day.

"Dr. McEwan sent me. To look at the incision," I responded.

I had on the patient gown with the front opening secured by two laces. Eager for medical attention I untied the straps, pulled the flaps apart, and exposed my chest the moment I finished speaking.

Since Dr. McEwan sent me to see him, they might have talked and the surgeon would be apprised of the purpose of my visit. The query "How can I help you?" was perhaps a ritual Dr. Shield had gotten used to and automatically replayed every time he met a patient. I was right. He did not follow my declaration with the usual questions a doctor would have asked if a patient had come with a new problem – What happened? When did it happen? How long had it been going on? He did not ask any of these questions. He did not even need any clarification before rendering his medical opinion as to the cause of the incision opening.

As if we were playing a game of surprises, I bared my chest without request or encouragement; in return he said something I never expected coming from a doctor.

"You're not wearing your bra."

I had been the ghostly inhabitant at home for more than a month, hardly moving, hardly making a noise, hardly thinking, and hardly feeling anything; his comment jolted me out of my semi-comatose state. Did my ears get it right? He was worried about what I put on? And of all things, my bra! The way he put it, he seemed to be referring not only to what I did not have on that day, but in the days past. He was pointing out what I wore or not wore at medical appointments and perhaps at all times.

In a television commercial an ophthalmologist tells her patient, "You have a disease called chronic dry eye." This happens on TV, not in real life; at least, not in my experience with doctors. After the initial choreographed performances explaining cancer and treatment, my interactions with my three doctors returned to "normal"; that is, the exchanges were curt and the encounters short. No one had told me my kind of cancer or my stage of cancer; no one had explained to me what happened when the incision opened or had spoken the word "seroma"; they only gave me instructions to follow. I only knew that something was leaking from my incision. Even in my ignorance, however, I had enough sense to catch what this doctor was saying. Like Dr. McEwan he had not looked at the incision, but he identified the cause of the leakage right then and there and blamed it on me. The incision opened because I did not wear a bra; a bra would have provided support and prevented the incision from tearing. I was responsible for what happened. It was my fault.

I brought it on myself! Ridiculous! Another case of blaming this victim! I thought of my friend who accused me of pushing the doctor to give me radiation before the incision was ready; she had not looked at the facts. And now this doctor jumped to a conclusion before examining the incision. What did my friend know? And now what did he know? How would he know if I wore a bra or not? I was in a patient gown every time I saw him, but I had to admit he was right. I did not wear one going to medical appointments because I had to strip; not having to take the bra off was easier on my debilitated arm and saved time. And how would he know I did not wear it at other times? I had to admit again that I did not. I had not worn one since surgery for the same reason of convenience. Still, it was none of his business and not something for him to say.

If a bra would support the breast and prevent the incision from tearing, why did he not tell me? If a bra could put pressure on the wound to stop fluid from accumulating or speed its dissipation if and when that occurred, why did he not warn me in the first place? He was the doctor; he should know and he should have told me. It was his job to alert the patient. I would have bandaged my chest around and around had I known it would help. At our first meeting I had asked him if I needed drainage – friends who had breast surgery had had a tube put in at the site to allow the fluid to escape; the surgeon answered no. Could it have been his oversight after all? Or could it be his error in judgment to give me glue not strong enough to hold the incision closed in the first place? The pectoral muscle in the chest is in action with every movement of the arm; perhaps he should have sewed and not secured the opening only with glue. Perhaps the usual one-month wait before radiation did not provide adequate time for an incision held together with glue to heal and the other doctor should have waited longer before radiating. He was blaming me, but he had to be blamed too.

When I mentioned to him in an earlier meeting in the week after surgery that my shoulder and arm hurt, he replied, "I did not cut the nerve." I did not expect him to say that and was taken aback by his quick response to absolve himself of his responsibility. I did not know that a severed nerve could restrict arm movement and cause pain. When I mentioned this to him, I was not thinking that something was wrong; I simply took the pain to be a normal fallout after the operation and was only seeking advice on how to alleviate the discomfort. The thought of holding him responsible never even crossed my mind.

He was not alone in being defensive. I asked Dr. McEwan casually at a follow-up meeting sometime after active treatment why she continued radiation when the incision opened. I was curious to know her reason, or perhaps I wanted to see how she would react. She told me Dr. Shield asked her to do it. That was the closest she came to admitting any responsibility for her action – she was following an order from the surgeon, and she blamed him. If medical friends hesitated to give me a diagnosis or recommendation on the opened incision without seeing me when I asked for advice, it would surprise me if the surgeon acted any differently; I had not seen Dr. Shield until she gave me the referral to do that. She was the expert in this kind of medical treatment, and it was also very unlikely that a surgeon would give advice to a radiologist to continue radiation. Continuing radiation was her decision, not the surgeon's. It takes courage to admit a mistake. Doctors are human, and they do not like to admit to making errors. They are especially quick to absolve themselves from any responsibility and blame each other if anything goes wrong in these litigious times. A court hearing would bring negative publicity and a negative court decision would bring harsher consequences, including a tarnished reputation, compensation or penalty to be paid, higher insurance costs, or even a suspended license; even an out-of-court settlement would be costly because they would have to pay indemnity and higher insurance.

Doctors try to protect themselves in other ways too. The radiation oncologist's report of our first meeting was a good example; it was in the file I obtained from the clinic. Dr. McEwan wrote in the report that she warned this patient that arrangement for radiation was tentative until surgery was done; she also put down that she told me I would not need radiation if I had a mastectomy. This is what a doctor following medical protocol will tell a patient; my recollection of the meeting was very different. She focused on the different kinds of radiation and tried to sell me hypofractionation; the word mastectomy never came up, and I left the meeting with the understanding that I was to return a month after surgery for radiation. After reading her report I checked with Victor to see if he heard anything different, but he had heard what I heard. If I were to sue her, as some patients might do, she would produce the document as evidence that she followed medical protocol by giving me all the information; returning to do radiation was my choosing. It would be her words and her written report against my words, my bad hearing, my thick skull, and my weak memory should litigation come to pass, and I would be furious to hear her say she did what she had not done. I did not sue her. The thought of doing that did come to mind, but I decided against it because it would be so painful to relive what happened.

Dr. Shield's statement on the absent bra was another example of a doctor's attempt to protect himself. To blame the opened incision on my sartorial negligence was his preemptive move to hold me responsible for what had happened. He was accusing me for no good reason. I recognized this even in my brain fog. If I were my old feisty self, or if I was feeling stronger, even my reticence to speak up or to take on doctors could not and would not hold me back. I would tell him he was wrong and why; I might even use the occasion to vent the pent-up frustrations of the last few weeks to hurl a few sharp verbal barbs at him.

Alas, I was not my normal self. I had lost much of the capacity to feel and the energy and ability to fight. My emotional reactions were not as strong or as intense as on the day Dr. McEwan sent me back to the radiation room. Dr. Shield was accusing me of something I did not deserve, holding me responsible for something that was not my doing; that shook me up. I was angry, but I was not angry enough, or I was not angry for long enough to get back at him. I was tired. My brain was not working properly, and I was not thinking clearly. The ideas did not go through my head in the way I had presented them here. Like bolts of lightning streaking across the sky, these thoughts emerged, surfaced in no particular order, flashed in every direction, were all over the place, disappeared as fast as they appeared, and reappeared or were never to be seen again, with some vanishing before I could even grasp them. If I were to articulate the thoughts in the way they were going through my head, they would come out muddled, making little sense and befuddling any listener. My arguments would be instantly dismissed as the incoherent ranting of an angry woman; I would not have been able to make my case.

Like the Arctic bear stirring from its deep sleep when the temperature warms up and the snow melts in spring, I was too groggy to feel, too confused to think, and too lethargic to give these emotions and thoughts expression. Like the bear feeling weak after starving all winter, I was exhausted and tired. To fight Dr. Shield would burn energy that I did not have and wore me out even more. I let it go and kept my silence. I did the right thing. I needed this doctor's medical attention, and he more than made up for his uncalled-for remark in the weeks to follow.

FIFTEEN

Safe at Last

Dr. Shield blamed the incision reopening on my sartorial neglect – I did not wear a bra to protect it. He was wrong, but I did not point this out to him. No one wants to offend his or her caregiver, especially when it is a doctor; the person wants to remain in the doctor's good graces. Besides, in a tug of war between the doctor and patient, without the doctor's expertise the patient usually loses. Didn't my tussle with Dr. McEwan turn out that way? If I had one with the surgeon, I would not be able to defend myself either; the result would be the same. Arguing with the surgeon would get me nowhere and bring me no benefit. I had learned my lesson. I did not respond to Dr. Shield's accusation and did not say another word. I accepted defeat silently if not graciously.

The surgeon asked me to go to the examination table so he could take a look at the incision. Someone was finally doing something about a problem that was neglected by the other doctor and had haunted me for so long, so I eagerly complied and climbed onto the table. He felt my breast and turned to the nurse for an applicator, the popsicle stick doctors use to depress the tongue and examine the larynx. The surgeon poked at the incision, and half of the six-inch probe went in. I felt and saw nothing; Victor told me what he did.

The two imperceptible pin-sized holes had dilated to connect and formed one big, gaping hole wide enough for the applicator to go in. It was good that I was too distraught in those last weeks of radiation to check the damage; it would alarm me too much to follow its progression. I did not need the additional worry; it would make me want to stop the treatment even more. I might not have the courage to confront the doctor, and not doing that would be more miserable. Even if I did take her on, I did not think she would listen and change her mind; I would be angry and again more miserable. Dr. McEwan wrote in her report that the incision was "almost healed when radiation ended"; again, what she wrote did not match the facts. She was very wrong. Clearly the incision had not healed. Anyway, how would she know? She had hardly given it a second look since the day she declared it ready for radiation.

I close my eyes when the dentist works on my teeth because I have no interest in staring at his goggled eyes or masked face. When he tilts the chair and my feet get higher than my head, blood rushes down into my brain, and I feel relaxed. Dr. Shield did not have the examination table tilted and my body remained level. Nevertheless, as soon as I felt his gloved fingers probing around the incision, I had the same surge of good feelings without the blood rushing to my head. It was a different type of feeling good. My agony, my anxiety, my anguish, and all my negative feelings evaporated. I stopped telling myself that treatment would kill. I stopped asking what was happening. I stopped wondering why it happened. I stopped worrying about the fall-outs. I even stopped thinking of cancer returning. My brain stopped racing.

If Michelle, the nurse, had picked this moment to check my vitals she would find my pulse slowed and my blood pressure returning to normal. I was calm. I took in one deep breath, filling my chest with oxygenated air, and exhaled slowly, pushing out the deoxygenated gas. My lids rested heavily over my eyes. My fists uncurled, my fingers straightened and felt the smooth paper under my palm on the examination table. My legs shifted slightly, my feet dropped a little, and the calf muscles loosened. In fact, the taut muscles all over my body unwound. I could have been meditating and the examination table my yoga mat. I had not been so much at ease, if not at peace, for a long time.

The opened incision no longer seemed to matter. Had I known at that moment that the tiny openings had expanded to create a gaping hole and that the applicator would go in I do not think I would feel any different from what I just described. A doctor was looking into the problem and fixing it; I was confident he would do his best and everything would come out right. I was not afraid or worried. The image of doctors as saviors in the world of disease has earned them adulation from a lot of patients; I respected doctors, though I had never given them the same degree of deference. Having been starved of medical attention for so long, I might be ready to do just that and give him the same deference in my gratitude for what he was doing. Even if I had not gone to that extreme, I became the trusting patient once more and perhaps a trusting patient as I had never been before.

I began to understand how quacks can take advantage of the sick who are desperate for a cure. A drowning person clutches at straws, any straw. When conventional medicine fails to provide the remedy, a patient who is fearful but does not want to give up hope searches for a cure. In such a situation it is easy to latch onto someone, anyone promising hope no matter how incredulous or preposterous the suggested treatment may seem to an observer. I am generally levelheaded. My medical condition was not urgent or terminal and I did not fear for my life, yet when the last doctor ignored me and did nothing, I felt so lost, so fearful, and so scared. I floundered and I flailed. When I was lying on the examination bed, I was more than ready to put my life into this doctor's hands and hung onto him. Luckily, this time my trust was not misplaced.

The surgeon did not open the incision and sew it back as Dr. McEwan had warned me earlier. He did not have to; the incision was already opened and he kept it open instead to let it heal from the inside.

"We cannot let it close. We have to keep it open or you may develop an infection, or worse, an abscess. We do not want that." He explained.

Dr. Shield might not have been the most articulate of doctors, but he had always been the most democratic, open, and transparent among the three looking after my breast cancer. From the start he gave me a choice between a lumpectomy or a mastectomy, assuming I would know the difference. He told me how he would take the tumor out and how he would close the incision. I might not always like his answers to my questions, but he always responded directly when I asked him anything. He was at it again with his version of a patient-centered approach. He described how he would close the wound and why he would do it that way; the pronoun "we" was especially sweet to my ears, because the plural suggested a collaborative effort; we were a team fighting the battle together. Of course, he would be the leader and I the follower, and I willingly accepted this subordinate role to follow his directions.

There is no one way to be patient-centered; there are a hundred and one ways to do so. A lot depends on what the doctor and patient bring with them into the examination room. Doctors have different characteristics and different personalities; they come from different cultures and family backgrounds, they have different life experiences, and the same goes for the patients. Each doctor feels comfortable with a different way of treating patients, and each patient with his or her individualized characteristics does not react in the same way to the same overture. It is not easy for doctors to pick the right approach, especially given the limited time the practitioner can spend with each. Even when the same two persons are involved, the "best" way to make the patient feel at ease rests on the kind of disease, the stage of the disease, the type of care required, and the person's mood on the occasion; the doctor has to be flexible and adjust his or her demeanor in each situation. This is not an easy task; however, the patient will usually appreciate the effort if the doctor tries. I might not have been 100 per cent satisfied with Dr. Shield's version of patient-centeredness, but I was happy when he showed his respect for me, treated me decently, and did his job responsibly.

The nurse opened a pack of sterilized gauze ribbon, and the doctor pressed the long strip into the opening, stopping only when he could go no farther. Again, I did not see this; Victor told me afterward. The medical profession labels the procedure "packing" and rightly so. It captures neatly what the surgeon was doing. He pressed or packed the gauze into the open wound to keep it from closing so the dead tissues and other unwanted materials could come out and make room for new growth; the wound would heal slowly from the inside before the opening closed.

When Dr. Shield finished "packing," he protected the opening with dressing and said, "Come back day after tomorrow." We lived some distance from his office, but I was more than happy to make the long trip that day and every day if necessary to put an end to a problem that had been dragging on for too long. I was grateful to have some-one paying attention to the problem. I visited his office three times that week and in the two weeks to follow.

Doctors have a way of quickly removing what they do not want patients to see; I witnessed that once before. The neu-rosurgeon asked my mother-in-law to sit up from her bed in the recovery room after radiosurgery. The procedure was somewhat like my breast cancer radiation, but it was a one-time operation sending beams of gamma rays to her brain tumor while her head rested on a pillow and had a square support clamped onto it. As soon as she lifted her head, I saw fresh red all over the pillow; I was not sure if the blood was from the clamps closing too tightly on her head or if it was a normal result from clamping. The doctor pulled the blood-stained pillow away with amazing alacrity – or perhaps "snatched" would be a better word to describe the action – and dumped it on the floor with the clean side up. He thought no one would notice, but I caught it all.

In the beginning weeks Dr. Shield asked me to lie down when he did his packing. He might have asked me to do this for the same reason the neurosurgeon dumped the pillow face down on the floor – he did not want me to see what he was doing or what was coming out of the wound. At the end of the second week, or perhaps the beginning of the third, he did not tell me to lie down. I sat on the examination table when he removed the dressing. The once-white gauze was covered with an abundance of minuscule dark particles layer over layer, reminding me of dead ants killed in their nest after being sprayed with a lethal insecticide.

"What's that?" I asked, curious to know more about these dead ants.

I was not the queasy type. I have always enjoyed watching medical shows on television and found medical documentaries interesting; the palpitating hearts and slippery livers inside the human body never fazed me.

"Granulation," the doctor answered, dumping the stained gauze into the trash can faster than he could utter the word.

Granulations are tissues and blood vessels formed during healing. The black debris on the gauze might have been granulation once, but now they were dead tissues expurgated from inside my opened incision, products of continued radiation and medical neglect. The proper medical term for these dead tissues is "eschar." Perhaps the surgeon used the word granulation to make it sound innocuous to the patient. He did not have to worry; I did not and would not know the difference until later, when active treatment was over. At the time, I only wondered how much of this gunk and what else might have come out when I was lying down.

The number of visits to Dr. Shield's office dropped from three to two times a week, and then to once a week. He did the packing in the first weeks and then stopped coming, perhaps, to quote Dr. McEwan, when the wound was "almost healed"; the nurse took over the task in his stead. Dr. Shield was nowhere in sight, but I trusted him and was not concerned. Ever since the day he started packing, I was confident that he would make sure nothing bad would happen. Just as in the last days of radiation, I did not check the incision; before it was because I was too distraught to do so, but now I had enough confidence in the doctor not to worry.

Dr. Shield reappeared in his blue scrubs on the last day of my visits, with Michelle trailing behind him. He checked the incision, now closed, and said, "You're all right. You don't have to come again. It's a long drive." This was good news; the doctor declared me whole. And he remembered where we lived and appreciated our efforts coming all the way to see him; really, I should be the one to thank him for taking care of me. These were my first thoughts. On second thought, I knew I could be wrong. He was telling me to stop coming, that I was dismissed. I appreciated his diplomacy just the same; he was being courteous. When I was angry with Dr. Shield's statement on the missing bra, I grudgingly gave him credit for his keen observation and good memory. After all that he had done for me in the past month and more I was ready to be generous and add to his list of strengths sensitivity and good bedside manners.

Michelle left the room with the doctor close behind her. He had his hand on the door, hesitated, and turned to face Victor and me. We had been coming so many times so regularly in the last little while that his stiff shell had softened somewhat. He no longer said, "How can I help you?" when he entered the examination room; he asked instead "How are you today?" and on the odd occasion he sighed and exclaimed, "Oh, it has been a busy day." Now this shy man looked at me, his brown eyes warm and friendly, and on his lips the faint smile I found so attractive in his internet photo. He said, "You are tough." The man in blue scrubs hardly finished the three words before he turned his back to us, reached for the handle a second time, and closed the door.

Did I hear him right? He never said much, but what he said could astound me. His earlier comment on the missing bra made me angry enough to shock me out of my daze. He surprised me again, this time his parting words shooting me up to cloud nine. He was complimenting me on how I handled the situation. I was strong! I was stoic! And I was resilient! He did not exactly say those words, but I quickly attributed these qualities to someone who was "tough." I could have pranced around in jubilation if I had the energy to do that, but I did not. I stared, mouth agape, at the closed door and then smiled.

Dr. Shield was not around when the incision opened. He never asked me what had happened or how it happened; he just worked on it. I did not offer him my side of the story either let alone share with him my anguish and agony in the weeks before he came onto the scene. We never talked about the ordeal. When he said I was tough I did not know if he was referring to how I took it before his appearance or since or in both times; it had been difficult when there was no one to turn to and it was easy once he was there to take care of the wound. It did not matter which period he was referring to; I took the comment as a compliment just the same. He showed his appreciation of what this patient had gone through and made me feel good to know that someone, a medical doctor, recognized my trials and appreciated my pain.

Those three words told me this doctor was sensitive, sympathetic if not empathetic, and supportive. He understood what I had been through. It would have comforted me so much to hear him say those words when the incision opened; hearing that would help so much in those difficult times. I would not have been so lost or felt so much anguish and so much pain. I had no doubt he would recognize the problem and would have done something if he had known; and if he did, I might have avoided the additional radiation, the incision would have closed a long time ago, and I might be well enough to be with Father in Hong Kong at this time. He came onto the scene a little late and he uttered those words a little late; nevertheless, I was happy to hear him say them just the same.

The doctor's words were a validation of what I had always thought and had wanted so much and for so long to hear someone say. Dr. Shield did not say it explicitly, but the message was clear enough. The incision opening was not a figment of my imagination, something I had made up even though the radiation oncologist treated it as such and ignored it. I had a medical problem serious enough to warrant medical attention; I had not exaggerated it. My worries were justified, the request for attention was reasonable, and my instinct was right – something should have been done about it at the time. The radiation oncologist was wrong to dismiss my concern, to ignore the opened wound and do nothing about it; her decision to continue radiation exacerbated the problem, and I paid the hefty price for her oversight, negligence, and neglect. The surgeon mended the wound, and his compliment regarding my toughness was an affirmation of what I had thought all along. I am not always right and do not have to always be right, but it was good that Dr. Shield agreed with me after the anguish I had been through. I felt vindicated.

The statement "You are tough" made me feel so good. The three words were the acknowledgment I had wanted so badly and for so long; it came unexpectedly from this quiet, laconic man and doctor. The three words he uttered was an encore to the music he played earlier in my ear to declare me whole, only it was much sweeter, more enchanting, and more exhilarating. He had just played me my personal Ode to Joy!

SIXTEEN

Another Lifeline

Dr. Gold, the medical oncologist, did not recommend chemotherapy for my treatment, but he asked me to return to get a prescription after I finished radiation. He did not tell me what the drug was, why I had to take it, or for how long. The web doctor told me this was adjuvant therapy to lower the chance of cancer returning. Patients usually take the medicine for five years after the active treatment phase; the particular drug taken depends on the type of breast cancer and the age of the recipient. Post-menopausal women like me with hormone-positive breast cancer take letrozole, an enzyme inhibitor, to stop and lower the production of estrogen that can promote the growth of cancer cells that may still be in the body; and younger women usually take tamoxifen, which targets the estrogen receptors of these cells to prevent their proliferation.

Dr. Gold did not offer me the information; he was not the only doctor to act this way; many doctors behave likewise.

Dr. Shield was perhaps one of the rare ones to explain to patients what he was doing. How many patients would think of asking doctors questions? Many would be too timid or too distraught with their ailments to do so; others would not know what to ask; only the very quick thinking, the informed, or those who know something about the subject may come up with questions. And some doctors would not answer even when patients do that. When I asked Dr. McEwan months later why the incision opened during radiation, she brushed me off, saying, "This sometimes happens." This was her answer, or non-answer; I did not learn anything from what she said. If I did not have a copy of her report, I would never have known anything about seroma or that she thought it was a possible cause.

Members in the cancer support group had similar experiences. A woman at the meeting was surprised to hear us talking about stages of cancer; she did not know there were stages in cancer let alone hers. Some doctors do not see it necessary to give patients information; perhaps they believe the knowledge will make patients worry. Some may think the patients are not interested in additional information, and others perhaps believe the patients will not understand. There may be a grain of truth in all these conjectures. From my experience, most patients do want to know what is wrong with their bodies. They may not understand the complexities of cancer or its cure, but they appreciate it when doctors use layperson's terms to explain what is going on. I am among this group. I do not care if doctors tell me what they do in their off-hours, but I do want to know about my medical condition and treatment.

The three cancer doctors treating me were trained in three different universities and spent their residencies in three different hospitals. If I were to include those looking after my comrades in the cancer support group, these alma maters spread all over the country, yet their graduates often seemed to behave in a more or less similar way as far as providing patients with information. They generally did not seem to see it necessary to explain to patients their medical conditions or the treatment they were to receive. Some doctors did not like getting questions; a good example would be the university clinic doctor who saw my curiosity to know more about allergies as distrust. And one member in the support group told an incredible story of how his doctor, who felt he was asking too many questions, told him not to speak until spoken to; even kindergarten teachers would not do that to their students.

I can only come to one conclusion. Even though connecting with patients is essential in effective medical practice, communication training may not have been a priority in many medical schools, or the students may not take learning these skills seriously when such courses are offered. Their focus is on imparting and mastering the science and know-how of healing, forgetting that doctors work with people and that effective communication with patients is integral to the practice of medicine.

I may be wrong; perhaps some doctors consciously or subconsciously see themselves as knowledgeable (which is true) and superior to patients and do not find it necessary to share information with or listen to the latter. They overlook the possibility that doctors who do not listen to patients may miss problems in their diagnosis and those who do not explain what they are doing may not get patients' full cooperation. The professional medical organizations recognize these problems and call on doctors to respect patients. If one respects a person, one listens and takes seriously what the other says and shares with the other person his or her thinking.

I saw Dr. Gold in January once radiation was over. He was sitting in front of the computer in his windowless office. Unlike the doctors in Hong Kong who are often cordoned off from patients with their huge, imposing desks, there was only an empty space between us, perhaps emblematic of the closer doctor-patient relationship in the West compared with the East. When I talked to a friend in Hong Kong about treatment, she comforted me, saying, "Do what the doctor tells you"; that is, everything would be all right if I followed the doctor's directives. Her unquestioning trust in doctors was typical of many other patients in Hong Kong and perhaps in North America too.

I had been quiet about the leaking wound; I did not tell my friends or even some of my family members because I did not want them to worry. Moreover, I did not like to repeat the same story over and over again; the telling and retelling fanned my anguish and increased my frustration, something I did not need. Most listeners would not understand what was going on and would ask more questions. I did not care to tell them, and I cared even less to explain; there was little they could do to help anyway. When friends asked how I was doing, I said everything was the same or changed the subject; when I felt very low with the continued radiation, I stopped picking up the phone and emailed them not to call.

Telling Dr. Gold was different. He was an oncologist and would understand what was going on without my elaboration. Besides, he was the doctor looking after me, and I had to keep him up-to-date on new developments. I poured it all out telling him what had happened in the last month.

The doctor listened intently, betraying no reaction as I recounted my story. When I came to the part about the incision opening, he leaned forward and nudged the side of the table with the palm of his hand; the chair moved forward and its four wheels slowed to a stop before it reached me. The doctor paddled the rest of the way with his feet until he faced me squarely. When I told him I tried to reference the American Cancer Society to get Dr. McEwan to stop radiation, Dr. Gold's eyes glinted and crinkled behind his dark-rimmed glasses; his upper lip lifted as if to break into a smile, stopped, and closed over the lower one to resume the subdued composure of a medical practitioner listening to a patient. He might have succeeded in holding back his amusement, but he could not contain his curiosity and cut in to ask for the result of my attempt before I could get to it.

"What did Dr. McEwan say?"

I had to report that my effort failed; I could not change the doctor's mind. He did not interrupt again until I ended my story.

"I was so confused and lost in the last couple of weeks. I did not know what to do." I probably looked that way too.

I stopped talking and expected the doctor to write the prescription for adjuvant therapy; but he did not.

"You should have come to me." He said instead.

The statement came as a surprise. It had never occurred to me to go to him on that agonizing weekend; my medical friend Stephen did not suggest seeing the medical oncologist when I asked him for advice. I had only seen Dr. Gold once at that time, and he was not involved in the surgery or radiation – that was my first thought and probably Stephen's reason for leaving him out. Almost immediately, I changed my mind. Perhaps I should have done that. Hadn't he spoken on my behalf with the blood testing company without my asking when he learned about the payment demand? He would have done the same and spoken to Dr. McEwan if he had known. He would have been my advocate on the matter, and I could not have had a better one. He would have asked the radiation oncologist to stop the procedure, as all my medical friends had said they would do. Dr. McEwan did not listen to me; she might have listened to her peers and I would have been spared of the ordeal.

His offer came a little late. The worst was behind me. Dr. Shield was working on the incision three times a week. I would not need his help.

"Dr. Shield is looking after the wound. I saw him yesterday and I'll go again tomorrow."

"From now on, call me whenever you have a problem."

Another proffer of help! A standing offer! A rain check! And from a medical doctor! Wow! He made the same offer twice; he was insistent! He meant it! What more could a patient ask for!

What a difference a day could make! Just the day before I was desperate for medical attention and did not dare raise my hopes even on the way to see the surgeon. I found help on Dr. Shield's examination table; now a standing offer of help from the medical oncologist! The ordeal was over. The nightmare in December seemed to be far away and so long ago. I could hardly remember how it felt, or perhaps I did not want to remember how it felt.

I had two doctors, one working on the physiological problem and the other offering emotional support and promising help if anything was to happen in the future! It was January and a new year; my luck had turned. I could have jumped for joy, but I was too weak. What had happened in the last month and more had drained my strength; my legs were too weak to lift me off the ground. In the excitement of getting help from another doctor my eyes sparkled for a split second, like the medical oncologist's a few moments ago, and I made a mental note to go to him in times of trouble.

I stopped short in my jubilation. At our first meeting Dr. Shield had asked me to call him anytime I needed help, but it turned out to be an empty promise because I could not reach him when I needed it. The surgeon's offer might have been a ritual statement made to patients, and if he did mean it, the staff in his office stood in the way. This might happen again. I believed Dr. Gold meant what he said, but there was no guarantee I could reach him through the office when the time came; I learned my lesson. I played cautious and "pushed" for a safeguard.

"Can I have your cell phone number just in case? It may be hard to reach you through the office."

I was stating a fact. Last September his receptionist would not let me see him when I called for an appointment; I had to wait until surgery was done. I had yet to learn that she was following medical protocol in cancer treatment – the oncologists work on the treatment plan (be it radiation, chemotherapy, or any other option or combination) only after the information is available after surgery and the second pathology report is out; any earlier plan is tentative, subject to change, and any earlier talks on the matter may be superfluous. On that day I did not know and still blamed the receptionist for blocking me access to the doctor for no good reason.

"I won't call unless it's an emergency and absolutely necessary," I told him.

The reassurance worked and he gave me his number. I kept my promise and never called him; I never had to.

Dr. Gold had no obligation to help me with the payment demand or the incision problem, let alone any future problems, yet he offered it just the same. He lived up to the image of the good doctor I picked up from the stories I read. He was the good doctor who cared for his patients; he would do what he could for them, would go out of his way to help, and would do more than was required without their asking. He was traditional in the way he dealt with patients; he did not initiate any social conversation or share with them his private life and focused instead on looking after his patients and having their interests at heart. I appreciated what he did for me, and I think his other patients could not miss the kindness behind his reserved demeanor.

I did not know what kind of help I would need from this doctor or what assistance he would provide in the future, but it did not matter. Patients trust doctors; I trusted this one. Doctors' medical expertise puts them in a special position in patients' eyes, and any offer of support from this quarter is especially appreciated. I knew his offer of help would not be an empty gesture and his promise not empty words. He had intervened on my behalf with the blood test company; I was sure he would do it again should the occasion require. His word was good enough.

Stress damages the body. When a person is under stress, the hormones adrenaline and cortisol spike, the heart pumps faster, and the blood vessels constrict. Prolonged exposure to high levels of these hormones leads to high blood pressure, insomnia, fatigue, and a myriad of other health issues. If the stress goes away soon enough, the body returns to equilibrium, metabolism returns to a normal level, and the fallouts from stress may disappear. If the stress remains for long enough, the health issues may stay and the damage becomes permanent. There is a strong link between the psychological and the physical, with one affecting the other.

Needless to say, a person diagnosed with breast cancer is stressed; any additional perturbation puts the patient's health at higher risk. Cancer worried me, the opened incision worried me more, and Dr. McEwan's insouciance and continued radiation worried me the most. I do not know what physical damages breast cancer and these additional stressors brought or if the damages stayed; I only know the distress had zapped my energy further and heightened my fatigue during this time. Once radiation stopped and the radiation oncologist was out of the picture, I felt relieved. I did not know if the damage went away with the stressor no longer there or if it stayed; I was tired and my energy remained low for a long time after.

When Dr. Shield "packed" the wound, he was doing something to mend the physical problem; his presence was a psychological boost as well. I became calmer, not as agitated as before. Dr. Gold's offer of help the day after I met the surgeon could not have been better timed or more opportune; he was giving me an additional lifeline. He did not do anything tangible, but he did not have to with the surgeon working on the incision. His assurance was a help just the same. I knew I would not be in a lurch should any problem come up in the future. He would be standing by to deliver effective help. I could count on him. I felt safe. My stress hormones probably went down with his gesture of support, his psychological remedy turning into a physical one.

I left Dr. Gold's office that January day without the prescription for adjuvant therapy; I had to come back when the incision closed. However, I did not leave empty-handed; I got something better – I had an assurance of help. And more than likely he would be my advocate, as the medical literature has always recommended and I had wanted so much in the last month. With help or the promise of help from this doctor, I became once more hopeful and confident that I could and would be well again. This assurance probably made for a faster recovery in the following two months than it would have been if it were not the case.

It is hard to isolate the effect of a drug or a treatment procedure on a disease in medical research; it is harder to document the impact of the psychological on the physical or vice versa and harder still to measure how much a particular treatment has contributed to a patient's recovery. The two doctors acted separately and in unison to bring me back to health. The gloom and doom I felt last December were replaced by hope in the new year; helplessness gave way to empowerment, desperation to relief, fear to courage, and darkness to light, and I could look forward to being well again. It would be difficult if not impossible to calibrate the benefits each doctor has brought me, but it does not matter how much each helped; I know both did and that was enough for me. If I had been teetering on the brink about to be swallowed by the gaping earth in the cancer seismic shift in those last days of radiation, the two doctors had pulled me away from the precipice to usher me onto the path to safety.

There are good reasons why commitment to warmth, sympathy, and understanding is integral to the Hippocratic oath taken by incoming doctors. The practice of medicine is largely self-regulated, with experts providing services to mostly uninformed patients who put their health, and in some cases their lives, in the hands of these practitioners. In the largely autonomous operation of the medical profession, the Hippocratic oath is the internal and internalized safeguard balancing the patient's well-being with the doctor's self-interest to ensure the latter will do the best for patients and not perform superfluous procedures let alone prescribe treatment that may harm the patient. Medical practitioners committed to these values are sensitive, quick to identify problems, prompt to provide remedies, and give timely, effective care. I am talking from experience. Dr. Shield and Dr. Gold were sympathetic, understanding, and warm; they gave me prompt, tangible remedies and much needed emotional support once they knew I had a problem. They were better doctors than the less caring one who let her patient languish.

The emphasis of the National Academy of Medicine and other medical organizations on patient-centered care offers another layer of safeguard to patients. This is all the more necessary with larger numbers of doctors working at private, for-profit medical organizations and coming under increasing pressure to "perform" and meet up to bureaucratic criteria that may conflict with patients' interests. The Hippocratic oath asks doctors to be committed to certain values, and the patient-centered approach focuses on their expressions. It reminds doctors of their fiduciary responsibility to serve patients, putting respect for and the needs of the patients in the forefront. If a person respects another, he or she listens to what the other says, is sensitive to the other's feelings, and does not ignore or peremptorily override the other's opinion; the doctor who respects the patient will take the patient's values, preferences, and needs into consideration when making clinical decisions.

After meeting with the two doctors, I could see the light at the end of the tunnel, the hope for recovery, and the possibility to be well again. I broke out of my catatonia of nothingness to notice things around me, to do things I had not done for a long time, and to turn to tasks that had been neglected. I watched the news on television after dinner only to fall asleep before it was over and learning little of what was going on in the world beyond. Once more I picked up the phone to reconnect with friends and kept the conversations short because I did not have the energy to talk longer. I wiped the countertop and neatly arranged the items on it; then I had a nap. I took out the towels haphazardly stuffed and squeezed inside the cupboard, folded them, and put them into a neat pile; then I rested in the afternoon. I became more ambitious and did more. I tidied a drawer in the kitchen, put the books back on the shelf, sorted the dated magazines on the coffee table, punctuating each job with breaks and following them with a long rest. Much to Victor's delight I put on the dining table the occasional Chinese vegetables, fish, beef, or chicken to break the monotony of the pork shank house special. And the jobs became more demanding as time went by. One day I threw away the leftover food in the fridge; my energy gave out before I could finish leaving containers dripping with condensation on the kitchen counter; Victor had to clear the mess. The number of unfinished tasks for him to complete multiplied, and if he did not get to it promptly enough, I reminded him. One day when I was a bit loud in prompting him to complete a task, he said in amusement, "You must be feeling better." The growing number of job orders and the frequent reminders became his gauge of my returning health.

Not everyone took these signals of recovery in such good humor. One March afternoon I was in Dr. Gold's office to pick up the letrozole prescription for adjuvant therapy. A few days earlier Dr. Shield had closed the incision and gave me the greatest compliment I had ever received from a medical doctor. I was in good spirits and believed I could be on my way to see Father soon. I was more talkative and pugnacious than I had been in a long time.

The doctor was perched on his stool, sending his prescription over the computer to the drugstore. His action gave me the idea and I said it out loud.

"I am taking letrozole for five years, I'll add to the success statistics."

As soon as the words came out of my mouth Dr. Gold's fingers froze over the keyboard like eagle claws hovering in mid-air ready to grip its prey; his upper lip closed over the lower one as if to hold back whatever he wanted to say. I could feel the tension from the dark silhouette of his face against the windowless wall. He remained motionless in front of the screen for what seemed to be a full minute before he pulled himself together to resume typing on the keyboard. When he finished sending the prescription, he turned coldly to me to issue a warning.

"Do not trust everything the web says."

In this age of information technology many patients, including me, scour the internet to learn about their diseases and treatment. We learn something, but we learn hardly enough to make a dent on the medical profession's monopoly of knowledge let alone to breach it. More often than not, what we learn from the web is simple, and in some cases inaccurate or outright wrong. Our incomplete knowledge, however, does stop us from speaking up and asking questions. This is a new problem for doctors to deal with. Some doctors may find it amusing, others see it as an opportunity to clarify and explain, and many more find it annoying, a pain, or an affront. I showed off my knowledge and Dr. Gold did not like it.

But what I said was true! I obtained the same information from multiple reputable sources. Cancer survival rate is usually measured by a patient living five years beyond the initial diagnosis. If I take the drug for five years and keep cancer away, I will be considered a case of success, a cancer survivor, and a success statistic! I was putting two and two together. My brain had started clicking after a long period of dormancy, an indication I was doing better. Dr. Gold did not appreciate this signal of recovery. He was not impressed with my insight or wit; instead, he seemed offended.

I forgot that doctors take their profession seriously, too seriously in my opinion. Their line of work high on the totem pole of professions is beyond the brunt of jokes even when these are generic ones not made at the doctor's personal expense. I should have known better than to be so flippant as to make such a facetious remark. Dr. Gold was the serious type. I should have gauged the listener before saying anything, especially when it was making light or making fun of something he cared so much about. It was obvious he took his work seriously; he cared a lot and did it well, just look at how he had treated me. I saw his response as overreaction, but I did not want nor did I mean to offend this good doctor who had done so much for me. His reaction alarmed me. I had not expected him to respond like this, and I had never seen him act like this. I was crestfallen and devastated, remorseful and repentant.

Dr. Gold was not only the serious type, he was cautious too. He asked me to stay around for another month to see him before leaving for Hong Kong. He did not give a reason why, and as usual I did not ask, but I could guess what he had left unsaid. He wanted to monitor my reaction to letrozole. He was doing his job and being careful. I appreciated his caution and acquiesced even though it meant another month's delay before I could see Father.

SEVENTEEN

Home Again

The closed incision did not leave the imperceptible scar I was hoping for; the site was more like a caldera after a volcanic eruption or a crater struck by a meteor from outer space, a trough about an inch in diameter, darker than the rest of the skin with a reddish rim around the edge. The passage of entry to remove the tumor was clearly detectable. There was another horizontal line under the skin across the breast leading to the nipple, reminding an observer of the vein feeding into the volcanic vent or perhaps a sewage pipe under the road. These marks paled and discolored over time but stayed; these blemishes, however, do not bother me. I have never had the seductive curves many women are blessed with. My breasts are small and have never been a source of pride or a major factor in defining my identity. Besides I am too advanced in years to care how they look.

I was more concerned to see Father in Hong Kong as soon as possible. I canceled the trip last September and postponed it to December, then it was moved from Christmas to Chinese New Year and I had to push it back again. I was more than six months behind my original date of arrival when I landed at the Hong Kong Airport in April. Ever since I told Father about the change of travel plans, I called him almost daily hoping the regular phone exchanges would allay his anxiety and assure him that I was doing all right. In December I was anxious when the incision opened, not knowing what was happening to my body; the experience taught me that not knowing was agonizing and could make a person imagine the worst. It was better to tell Father something than to keep him completely in the dark or he might conjure up the worst scenario to explain my absence.

When I could not go at Christmas, I could not blame Victor for the delay as I had earlier; it would not be fair to scapegoat him a second time, and no one would believe it anyway. I was not good at making things up. It was hard enough to come up with the first excuse in September, and to drum up another was almost impossible. I told Father the truth, or at least part of the truth. I told him about my breast cancer and what I thought was adequate – that it was early-stage breast cancer and that I had to stay behind for treatment – without mentioning the difficulties I was going through. I reminded him that cousin Theresa had recovered from her breast cancer to live a normal life and said I would be in Hong Kong for Chinese New Year.

I felt more relaxed after telling Father about my illness because I did not need to be so vigilant when talking to him on the phone. He seemed satisfied; he did not ask how treatment was going nor how I was doing in our almost daily phone conversation. The lack of inquiry did not mean he did not care; I knew he did, he just did not know what to say. Like me in medical offices, perhaps he did not know what to ask. Or perhaps my almost daily call assured him that I was doing all right; I hope the last was the case. And more than likely, he knew me well enough to know I would not tell him any more than what I had offered; it was useless to ask because he would not get a straight answer. He was right; I would not tell him what I was going through because I did not want him to worry.

Our almost daily conversation over the phone was short, artificial, and a little forced. While we both enjoyed hearing from the other, we had little to say; there was nothing going on in our lives that we cared to share or found interesting enough to be worth mentioning. We spent most of our time resting and doing nothing. Our conversations were mundane, bordering on the boring. We reported on the minutiae of what we did that day, which was not much, or what we ate, which was even less exciting. However, if we did not talk about those very boring subjects, we would have nothing to say to each other.

Chinese New Year fell on February 19 on the Western calendar; the day came and went. Dr. Shield was working on the incision, and I could not leave town with the open wound. I stopped giving Father a reason for the delay and just said I could not come back just yet. I promised to be there by March; with Dr. Gold wanting to monitor my reaction to letrozole, the visit was pushed back again for another month to April. Father accepted the change of dates every time without a murmur; however, he told his physiotherapist, who in turn told me when I was in Hong Kong, that he was very disappointed with my absence in the Chinese New Year. He said I promised to be there for the occasion and did not keep my word. Chinese New Year, like Christmas in North America, is the most important family holiday of the year.

Cancer treatment took twice as long as I had expected. I was in Hong Kong two months after Chinese New Year and more than six months behind my original scheduled arrival date. Father was excited to see me. In the first week of my return, he wanted to do all the things we used to do when we were together. He suggested going to a movie. It was one he picked, an action movie not exactly to my taste, but I went just the same. I could not remember the title, nor did I have a clue about the plot. He enjoyed it, and that was what was important. We went to Dragon Inn, his favorite dim sum place, to enjoy his coveted Chinese dainties: shrimp dumplings, pork suimai, spring rolls, and fried noodles. Like people of his generation who suffered through the lean years of the Second World War, he said the price was too high and the restaurant was gouging, but it did not stop him from savoring the food. He loved being outdoors, but his lack of strength and mine could not take us far. In the past we would have taken the ferry for a day trip to one of the neighboring islands; this time we remained on the main one and took a taxi to Victoria Park with its botanical garden, swimming pools, ball courts, and soccer fields, not far from the apartment. Father sat in his wheelchair looking through the chain-link fence at the two tennis players on the court. His stationary head and somber expression told me he was not following the game; he was reminiscing about the time when he played and wished longingly to do it again. Early another morning we strolled along the waterfront to avoid the strong sun later in the day. He wanted to sit on the bench; Winnie parked his wheelchair at an angle to it, and together we helped him up, rotated him forty-five degrees, moved him back a few steps until his legs touched the edge of the seat, and he sat down. The strenuous transfer was well worth the effort; to see him sitting contentedly on the bench like any park visitor sipping from a small carton of soy milk and taking in the cruise ships, freight boats, tankers, ferries, yachts, and sampans that were gliding across the waters reminded me of the good old days.

Father was excited with my coming, his adrenaline flowed; the spike of energy, however, could not last forever. He was much weakened since my last visit and found it difficult to walk the thirty-odd steps from the apartment door to the building elevator. Pain in his belly had spread to his chest, and he could hardly move his arm; he blamed the pain in his arm on the physiotherapist making him work too hard. He took stronger painkillers, and more frequently, which made him groggy. Before the week was over his body would not cooperate; the excursions had to stop. Father went back to his routine of staying indoors and sitting in his wheelchair all day every day. He would make the few essential steps to get into bed or go to the bathroom with Winnie's help; otherwise, he remained in the wheelchair, even for meals. His appetite had diminished; he chewed his food slowly and swallowed with difficulty. He did not say as much as he used to, which had never been much anyway, and answered in monosyllables if I asked him anything. He no longer watched the replays of old movie classics in the afternoon or stayed up for the primetime programs on television in the evening. He spent a lot of his time dozing in the wheelchair or lying on the bed. His daily routine suited me, because I did not have the energy to do much either; when he rested, I did the same.

All the while in Hong Kong I had the feeling it might be the last time I would see him. When I was to leave, Father did not offer to see me off at the airport, something he had always done every time I visited. Going to the airport was something he had always enjoyed. The air terminal was not as crowded as the streets; its flat surface offered him an easier place to walk compared to the uneven street pavement and its many potholes. In the early years after his stroke he hobbled along, holding a cane in one hand and the helper holding his other arm; as he grew weaker over the years we took his wheelchair along so he could sit if he got tired. We would spend a few leisurely hours in the terminal to window shop and grab something to eat, then I would put him on the bus or a taxi to go home if he would let me before I boarded the plane.

On the morning of my departure, I went into his room to say goodbye. He had exchanged his bed against the wall for the hospital bed in the middle of the room to make it easier for someone to help him. The sun was blinding outside; his face remained in the shadows, shaded from the strong sun by the headboard with its back to the window. When I came to where he was lying, he whispered slowly and with some effort.

"I love you very much; you don't know it."

His words came as a complete surprise; it was not his usual farewell. In the past he would tell me to take care, to come back soon, and to come back often. He had just said something a Chinese man of his generation would rarely or never say to his children – to proclaim their love for their child. The cohorts of his age usually kept their emotions to themselves; the only exception was perhaps anger when they released their pent-up frustrations at their wives, children, and subordinates in their bad moments. Father did not exactly fit this profile; he was easy-going, happy-go-lucky, and laughed a lot. Nevertheless, he kept his feelings to himself. He never complimented us as children and never once said he loved us. This was his first affirmation of love for his daughter, and sad to say his last too.

His action took me by surprise, but the message did not. Of course I knew. I knew it all along! How could I not? He loved me and he loved my brothers! He might not have put his feelings for his children into words, but he had shown it in more ways than one, many times, and all the time. I felt it every time I was in Hong Kong, whether I was the young adult, the middle-aged woman, and now the senior. I felt protected, pampered, and perhaps a little spoiled. I might be annoyed when he reminded me to dress warmly before going out, but I knew he cared. I only had to mention I had not tasted some Chinese delicacies for a long time and the dish would appear on the table the next day. He loved me, and very much! Despite the patriarchal Chinese culture that emphasizes male dominance, fathers still have a soft spot for daughters, and I was his only one. My brothers recognized this even when we were young; they made me go to him for things they were too afraid to ask for or thought they might not get if the request did not come from me. This special place I enjoyed among my siblings did not stop me from accusing Father of subscribing to the Chinese tradition to value sons more than daughters and caring for my brothers more than me. I knew this was not true, but that did not stop me from saying it to his face when I was young, perhaps as retaliation when he reprimanded me for misbehavior; all these years I teased him, repeating the same accusation again and again. I did not mean it; I never said it with a straight face. I did it out of the pleasure to see him annoyed and watched his discomfort. When I teamed up with my younger brother to accuse Father of subscribing to primogeniture, doting on my older brother more than us, it was sheer fun. My older brother did have a special place in his heart. Firstborn children usually steal their parents' hearts, but that did not mean he loved us any less. With two against one, we put Father on the spot and he was at a loss for words; I was gleeful.

Now I know I was cruel. I was the bully inflicting suffering on another out of fun, and the victim was my own father. I hurt him then and now it hurt me. I never thought Father would take it so seriously and so much to heart. He knew he did not have much time to live and had to make his love for me clear. He did not want me to go on living thinking I was any less loved than my brothers. He wanted to assure me of his affection even when it took him so much effort to say those words. He loved me so much! And I had been so cruel! I could not shake off the thought that what

I said had weighed on him so much and for so long. The accusations said as a joke had made him feel bad and stung him sharply. I should not have been so insensitive; I should not have poked fun at him. I should not have said it so often and so many times. It pained me to realize what I had done.

Tears swelled in my eyes and I wanted to cry. I did not want him to see me like that. Seeing me leave was bad enough; it would cause him more pain to see me upset. I wanted to repeat those same words he had just said, "I love you too," but I could not bring myself to do it. I would not be able to finish the sentence; I would choke before the four words came out of me. I wanted to hug him, but I could not reach him lying on the bed with the railings rolled up. For a sixty-seven-year-old woman to hold her ninety-four-year-old father in her arms would break a centuries-long Chinese tradition. I was shackled to traditions and did not have his courage to defy convention, so I hesitated. I wanted to hold his hand, but I held back because to do so would signal a last farewell and give away my fear of losing him; I could not bring myself to do it. I could not bear to meet his eyes because I did not want him to see the tears coming out from mine. I looked at the wall with tears rolling down my face and said quietly, "I'll come back for Christmas," setting a date for our next meeting as I did every time before leaving; only this time I knew full well the emptiness of the promise, and he probably knew it too. I missed my chance to tell him how much I loved him. The following Saturday, he had breakfast, passed out, and passed on. Father died a week after I left.

EIGHTEEN

Epilogue

The six months of cancer treatment were the darkest days in my life; the last days of radiation were the worst, and I hit rock bottom with Father passing on. I did not bounce back to my normal self as fast as most women with early-stage breast cancer do. Three years later I am stronger than when I was going through treatment but not as strong as I was before the illness. I do not have the same energy or stamina; I get easily tired and need more frequent and longer rests. Instead of completing the weekly house cleaning in one go, I do one room at a time and rest in between tasks. Putting dishes back into the kitchen cupboard no longer takes the strenuous effort it did after surgery – my left arm does not need to hold my right elbow to complete the task – but my right arm is still too weak to lift cast iron pots or cookware filled with food. I stand at the kitchen counter to prepare food and at the stove to cook, but I need a stool if the task takes longer than five or ten minutes. The quick dinners I used to pull together in less than an hour have turned into two-to-three-hour projects, and preparation is sometimes split into segments during the day. Apart from dealing with these essentials of everyday living, I have little time or energy left to do anything else.

Four-hour hikes have shrunk to twenty-minute walks in the neighborhood; a longer walk requires the support of a hiking pole or cane. My shoulder pain subsided after a few months of physical therapy, but it has not disappeared for good; one wrong move can trigger its return. My right arm has a wider range of motion than when I was undergoing treatment, but I have to move slowly to prevent the pain from returning or further injury. My favorite front crawl in the pool is replaced by the breaststroke, which is easier on the arm but is not the kind of swimming I care for. Kayaking, badminton, tennis, and other more vigorous sports or outdoor activities I used to enjoy are out of the question.

I have not received chemotherapy, a treatment procedure that may affect the brain, but my brain is a little fried just the same. I have caught myself pouring tea into the cup over the spoon instead of the strainer, returning cutlery to the fridge instead of the drawer, and heading into a room only to stop and ask what I am going in for. I had once prided myself with photographic memory, now I have difficulty registering new information, recognizing and remembering faces, or recalling names and events. I stop mid-sentence, failing to find the word for what I want to say. Multitasking is out of the question because I make mistakes if I do. I know I will never be my old self again.

The loss of mental acuity and my weakening body may have something to do with my cancer or treatment, but age may be a contributing factor too. After all, I am not getting any younger; when readers read these pages, I will have become a septuagenarian. Many seniors at my age feel their weakening muscles, gnawing joint pain, drop in energy, and diminishing stamina; others become slow and forgetful without going through cancer. The decline in physical strength and brain power comes sooner or later with age; this is a law of nature that no one can escape. I am only lucky I did not suffer from these symptoms earlier; cancer and treatment have released their onset or accelerated the imperceptible downhill slide to remind me of mortality with more years behind me than ahead.

Most cancer patients are at a loss when they hear the diagnosis. Most know little about the illness, the treatment procedures, or the ins and outs of the medical system. I was among this majority. I was ignorant of the disease and treatment with the inadequacy compounded by an impatient personality and the urgency to be with a dying father. Together these made me more vulnerable to missteps. I made many mistakes in the course of seeking treatment and paid the price.

There is one important lesson I learned on this cancer journey, though, and perhaps it is something all cancer patients should take note of – patients have to be patient. When a person knows that she has breast cancer, it is natural to be anxious and eager to start treatment as soon as possible. However, she has to remember that the initial biopsies and tests do not tell the whole story; much-needed and more accurate information comes after surgery is done. This is why the medical treatment protocol recommends that a treatment plan be drawn up only after the tumor is taken out and the second pathology report is available. An experienced doctor may tell the patient what to expect; what is said remains a projection and may change. Scheduling radiation or chemotherapy (with a few exceptions) without this report in hand is generally premature; the patient has to wait for the pathology report to come out after surgery before committing to any action. I do not know the origin of the word "patient" to describe a person undergoing medical treatment; perhaps it was to be a reminder to those afflicted with any disease to practice patience.

Breast cancer patients will benefit from having an advocate by their side during this difficult time. The presence of a confidant will make the patient feel less stressed, less anxious, and calmer. This person lends another pair of ears in the examination room and can fact-check what the patient thinks she has heard. Outside the medical office, this person is a sounding board to hold back reckless decisions, dampen impetuous moves, and provide judicious advice. Should the situation arise, this person can add another voice to the patient's championing her wishes so they will be taken seriously by the healthcare providers. The advocate can be a trusted friend; if this friend is knowledgeable in medicine and familiar with the workings of the healthcare system, all the better; he or she can clarify reports, offer expert advice, and point to ways to get medical help.

In the course of cancer treatment, I came across kind and not so kind doctors, helpful and not so helpful professionals;

I am in no position to speak on their medical expertise, but I can appreciate the psychological differences a kind and caring healthcare provider can make on a patient. My experiences put me solidly behind the patient-centered approach advocated by the medical associations; a doctor with the patient's interest at heart is kind and caring. Doctors have personal interests and can come under conflicting pressures; the call for a patient-centered approach with the patient's interest put front and center offers a strong counterweight to such pressures that may undermine their commitment to patients.

Patient-centeredness singles out the need for doctors to respect patients and to take patient preferences into consideration in making medical decisions; I can attest to the adverse consequences when a doctor does not do that. Dr. McEwan ignored my wishes to stop radiation when the incision opened and continued treatment. She did not listen to me and ignored what I said. She did what she did without explanation and made light of the possible consequences. Her attitude and behavior upset me, making me feel worse in an already difficult time, and sad to say, her decision went contrary to what medical practice would generally suggest. The incision opened completely and the treatment time more than doubled.

The medical associations want doctors to give patients due regard, not high esteem when they ask them to respect patients. Doctors are to treat patients as equals, to be polite, to listen, and seriously try to see the latter's point of view. To me, this is a version of the caring doctor in a democratic age, a correction to the haughty attitude among some caring professionals of the past. When a doctor treats me with respect, I open up to tell my problem and cooperate with the directives. When I feel the other party treats me as inferior, I close up; that does not facilitate the healing process. Apart from listening to the patients, doctors can demonstrate patient respect in two active ways – explain to the patients what they are doing and answer the patients' questions. I make these suggestions based on my reactions to doctors' behavior. When Dr. Shield described how he would take the tumor out and what he would do to close the incision, I felt comfortable because I knew what was to come. Dr. McEwan attributed the leaking incision to seroma, I discovered that in her report, yet she would not tell me when I asked. I felt she considered me incapable of understanding the explanation or she was being dismissive by brushing me aside; I was hurt. Being open and transparent is a sign of respect; it helps to promote rapport between doctors and patients and puts the patient at ease.

There are many ways to demonstrate respect for patients; this is to be expected. With so many factors coming into play in any interaction, there is no one set way to do it. Different doctors use different strategies, they adopt different methods with different patients, and they vary their behavior in different situations, even with the same patient. There are many versions of patient-centeredness. Those of Dr. Shield and Dr. Gold could not have been more different; if I could summarize each doctor's approach in one word, one was open and the other reserved; yet they shared one thing in common – a strong sense of responsibility to bring the patient back to health, and Dr. Gold's commitment to the patient in particular went beyond the call of duty.

This commitment to the patient's welfare is fundamental in respect for patients and underpins patient-centeredness. To be patient-centered is not just being nice to the patient; doctors have to be compassionate and responsive to patient needs. Without a genuine concern for the patient's well-being, the pleasant behavior is superficial, no different from some traveling salesman sweet-talking and peddling his wares to customers with the latter's interests readily compromised when the tests come.

Having cancer once does not mean the person is immune from the disease; cancer may come back. Like volcanoes spewing lava and gas after a long period of dormancy, cancer in remission may come back; in fact, getting it once may suggest a higher-than-average probability that it may happen again, and if my suspicion that the incision reopened from an overdose of radiation is correct, the chance of cancer returning may be even higher. The damage is done if it has been done, and there is not much I can do about it. Like the inhabitants in an earthquake zone, I have to live with the predicament, not worry too much, and wish it will be a long time before cancer will recur and hope it will never return. If and when it comes back, I will try to remember what I have learned on this cancer journey to be patient and not rush into action. I will recruit an advocate, and with this person by my side I hope to make judicious decisions to avoid making the same mistakes a second time.

In the meantime, I accept the new normal with all its limitations. Christianity encourages the faithful to count their blessings; Islam believes that difficulties and hurdles come with living in this world; Buddhism and other Asian religions urge their followers to take things as they come. They seem to be talking about different things; the semantics may be different, but the essence of the message is the same – there are things beyond a person's control, so be accepting. I may not be a follower of Christianity or any of these religions; I can see that a person has to accept what is not in her control and be content or, to use a Christian term, to feel blessed with what she has. Dwelling on mishaps, complaining of losses, or blaming others for things gone wrong is counterproductive; this will only make the person feel miserable and those around feel bad. I shall not fret about what I have lost or complain about things I can no longer do. My health has come back, albeit not to the same level as before. I have my family and friends and enough resources to get by. I should treasure what I have and be content. Or in the contemporary diction, be grateful.

Acceptance is not to be passive; it is not my nature to do nothing. I will be active, enjoy the tasks I can do, and not get frustrated with what I can no longer do. I will do my best to face the challenges, to recognize my limits, to overcome hurdles, and to push new boundaries. Even if I fail in one or another of these endeavors, it does not matter, no harm is done. I gain new experiences, acquire new insight, and learn new skills through trials and errors.

I do not have to look to religion for inspiration or to look far for the benefits of this approach; I only have to look to my father. He did not become a recluse after a massive stroke that took away the use of his left arm and crippled his left leg. For the next twenty years and more he stayed active, exercised, and kept as normal a schedule as possible and enjoyed his life. When terminal cancer further weakened his body and he knew the end was closing in, he seldom complained. He continued doing things with his family and friends when his energy permitted and let them know he enjoyed every moment he spent with them.

My father's cancer brought him to his eventual end, something not surprising for a man in his nineties suffering from cancer. I miss him. Impatience to see him and to be with him made me act impulsively, almost giving up local treatment to seek medical help in a place I was no longer familiar with, and worrying about him had added considerable agony to an already difficult struggle with cancer. On the other hand, recalling how my father handled cancer in those last years of his life, when he knew his end was drawing near, probably kept me afloat in the darkest moments and rescued me from the deep abyss of despair I might otherwise have fallen into and never gotten out of. His example will continue to be my beacon in the years to come. He was not a hero in a society valuing money, accomplishments, and fame; he was an ordinary man with no stellar career or great worldly achievement, but he is my hero. His stoicism and tenacity in his struggle with cancer and his ability to enjoy the small things in life despite his physical disabilities and limitations have earned him my respect, and my own battle with cancer only brought home sharply the lessons he taught by example. He will continue to inspire me.

I went through a difficult cancer journey, and so did my father. Our two journeys overlapped and intertwined, and they ended very differently. I traversed the difficult cancer terrain to cross the phantom pass and look to the vista of health and living. I reach safety to enjoy my golden years, euphemism for the last stage in life with all its challenges. There will be more difficulties and new problems ahead; I am realistic. They will require innovative strategies and solutions. But I have learned from my cancer experience and from Father to become wiser and more prepared. Like Father, I will remain optimistic and stay upbeat to meet what comes on this next leg of life's journey. I will try to live up to being the daughter of the man with a zest for living.

Bibliography

Allison, Kimberly. *Red Sunshine*. New York: Hatherleigh, 2011.

Boyer, Anne. *The Undying*. New York: Farrar, Straus and Giroux, 2019.

Christakis, Nicholas A., and James H. Fowler. *Connected*. New York: Little Brown, 2009.

Edwards, Elizabeth. *Saving Graces: Finding Solace and Strength from Friends and Strangers*. New York: Random House, 2006.

Fox, Renee. *The Sociology of Medicine*. Englewood Cliffs, NJ: Prentice Hall, 1989.

Freidson, Eliot. *Professional Dominance: The Social Structure of Medical Care*. Chicago: Aldine Publishing Company, 1970.

Hartmann, Lynn C., and Charles L. Loprinzi. *The Mayo Clinic Breast Cancer Book*. Intercourse, PA: Good Books, 2012.

Kalanithi, Paul. *When Breath Becomes Air*. New York: Random House, 2016.

Lorde, Audre. *The Cancer Journals: Special Edition*. San Francisco: Aunt Lute Books, 1997.

Love, Susan M. *Dr. Susan Love's Breast Book*. Boston: Da Capo Press, 2010.

Makary, Marty. *Unaccountable: What Hospitals Won't Tell You and How Transparency Can Revolutionize Health Care*. New York: Bloomsbury Press, 2012.

Marsh, Henry. *Do No Harm: Stories of Life, Death, and Brain Surgery*. New York: St. Martin's Press, 2014.

Mukherjee, Siddhartha. *The Emperor of All Maladies: A Biography of Cancer*. New York: Scribner, 2010.

Munster, Pamela N. *Twisting Fate: My Journey with BRCA – From Breast Cancer Doctor to Patient and Back*. New York: The Experiment, 2018.

Novack, Nancy, and Barbara K. Richardson. *I Am with You*. Point Richmond, CA: Bay Tree Publishing, 2015.

Parsons, Talcott. "The Sick Role and the Role of the Physician Reconsidered." *Health and Society* 53, no. 3 (Summer 1975): 257–78. https://doi.org/10.2307/3349493

Raz, Hilda. *Living on the Margins: Women Writers on Breast Cancer*. New York: Persea Books, 1999.

Shapiro, Marla. *Life in the Balance: My Journey with Breast Cancer*. Toronto: Harper Collins, 2006.

Sherman, Kenneth. *Wait Time: A Memoir of Cancer*. Waterloo: Wilfrid Laurier University Press, 2016.

Sontag, Susan. *Illness as Metaphor*. New York: Farrar, Straus and Giroux, 1978.

Starr, Paul. *The Social Transformation of American Medicine*. New York: Basic Books, 2017.

Tennyson, Alfred. "The Charge of the Light Brigade." 1854. https://www. poetryfoundation.org/poems-and-poets/poems/detail/45319

Wadler, Joyce. *My Breast*. New York: Pocket Books, 1997.

Websites

www.breastcancer.org (Living with Breast Cancer)

www.cancer.gov (National Cancer Institute)

www.cancer.org (American Cancer Society)

www.drsusanloveresearchfoundation.org (Dr. Susan Love Research Foundation) Sherman, Kenneth.

www.komen.org (Susan G. Komen)

www.stopbreastcancer.org (National Breast Cancer Coalition)

Index

adjuvant therapy, prescription for,
    201, 210, 213
adrenaline, 138, 209, 221
advocate: benefits of, 230;
    doctor as, 206, 210; friend
    as, 230; patients as own, 156;
    private healthcare system, 114;
    recommendations for, 170–1;
    recruiting, 233
ageism, reverse, 75
alcohol, 59
American Cancer Society, 20, 21,
    24, 114, 154–7, 205
American Psychiatric Association,
    criteria for depression, 87
attitude, illness and, 103–4
authority, questioning of, 49

bacitracin zinc, ointment, 173
biopsy, breast, 9
biopsy report, 50, 62; clinical, 51;
    pathology, 51
Black Lives Matter movement, 180

blood pressure: hypertension, 54;
    pre-surgical, 71
blood test, 37, 58, 107–8; company,
    110, 111, 206, 209
brachytherapy radioactive
    materials, 119
brain, chemotherapy and, 228–9
brain fog, 91, 95, 108, 187
brain tumor, PET scan, 113
BRCA1 gene, 66
breast: biopsy, 9–10; cyst removal,
    6; lumps, 6; mammography,
    6–7; sonogram, 8–9; tagging
    the nodule, 10
Breast Book (Love), 20
breast cancer, 20–1; American
    Cancer Society recommenda-
    tions, 154–7; desire for a dream
    team, 39–40, 148; diagnosis
    of, 53, 143, 209; family history
    of, 66; foreshock, shock and
    aftershock of, 144–5; googling
    search term, 20; Hong Kong

breast cancer (*continued*)
treatment questions, 26–7;
incidence, 21–2, 25; letrozole
for hormone-positive, 201;
lobby, 22; medical protocol for
treatment, 52–3; medical science
and, 80–1; patient's journey,
229–32, 235–6; pronouncement
by doctor, 12, 14, 18; reaction
to, 19–20; shopping aerobics
and, 137–8; stage, 21, 24, 51, 66;
test for gene predisposing, 107;
treatment, 14–15; treatment
requiring specialists, 35–6; types
of cells, 21; worries about, 54–5;
X-ray radiation, 119
Breast Cancer Book (Mayo Clinic), 20
Breastcancer.org, statistics, 25
Brown, Dr. (pseudonym), surgeon, 36, 51
Buddhism, 233

Canada, 20; breast cancer rate, 21;
public healthcare, 115–16
cancer: "curing," 37; description,
20–1; diagnosis, 13, 23–4, 229;
dirty word, 10; Father's battle,
60–2; journey of, 235–6; questioning causes of, 59–60; questioning
"why me," 60; survival rate,
214–15; term "in remission," 23,
26; treatments, 22–4, 37–8;
treatment taking over daily life,
58; *see also* breast cancer
"cancer free," 23
Cancer Research Institute, 20
cancer society, support group of,
91–3
cancer specialists, 39; interactions
with offices of, 39–47
"cancer survivor," term, 25
Casodex, 13
catheter 61; infection, 4

Chang, Dr. (pseudonym), 1–5
"Charge of the Light Brigade,
The" (Tennyson), 159, 161
chemotherapy 228; brain and,
228–9; cancer treatment, 22–3;
experiences of others, 55–6;
scheduling of, 230; side effects,
55; surgery and, 68
chicken pox, 26
Chinese: culture 70; importance of
family, 7; language, 4, 9; medicine, 18; questions about name,
40, 44, 46; tradition, 223–5
Chinese New Year, 218, 219–20
Christianity, 233, 234
chronic dry eye, television commercial on, 183–4
cigarette smoking, 59
Cipro, 2
Clinton, Bill, 151
communication: changes in
couple's, 57–8; everyday living,
57; friends, 93–5; interacting
with medical offices, 39–47;
medical training institutes,
203–4; questioning on
experiences of friends, 55–6;
sensitivity in, 168–9
coping strategies, support group,
91–3
cortisol, 209
Covid pandemic, 97
CT (computerized tomography)
scan, 58
culture: British, 73; Chinese, 70, 73;
Chinese belief on knowledge
of old, 75; Chinese tradition,
224; Chinese upbringing for
obeying hierarchy, 158; nurse-
patient interactions and, 69–71

daily routine, 53, 57, 172, 222
death sentence, 2, 113

depression, 87, 172
diagnostic radiologist, surgery, 74–6
doctors: being patient-centered, 193–4; blaming the victim, 147–8, 184, 185; cancer treatment, 230–1; information technology and, 214; offering information to patients, 201–4; patient-centeredness of, 231–3; profession, 215; respect for patients, 231–3; self-protection of, 183–8
Do No Harm (Marsh), 72, 120
dream team, desire for, 39–40, 148

Edwards, Elizabeth, 90
elephant arm, 139
emotions, floodgates of, 59
Emperor of All Maladies (Mukerjhee), 20
exercise: daily arm, 130, 138, 139; independence, 131–2; mall walking, 130, 132–5; neighborhood walks, 228; "shopping aerobics," 137–8
external radiation beams, 118, 119

family doctor, 37; importance of, 7
Fata, Farid, fraud, 110–11, 160
Father: April Hong King visit to see, 218–25; cancer journey, 235–36; care in Hong Kong, 115; cheerful in last days of his life, 102–3; death of, 225, 227; delay of trip to see, 29–32, 127, 173–4; inspiration of, 234–5; live-in caregiver, 30–1, 61–2, 221; memories of good times with, 84; prostate cancer in, 2, 3, 5, 13, 61, 235; saying goodbye, 222–5; stroke, 30; terminal diagnosis, 5, 235; visit possibility, 198

fatigue, sleep and, 84–5
food: advice for nutritious, 96–100; juicing, 99–100, 101–2; pork, 97, 98; social culture and, 95–9
Ford, Betty, 22
Freidson, Eliot, 38
French Revolution, 163
friends, phone calls from, 93–5

Galleria Mall, 130, 132, 171
gender equity, 180
girl, descriptions of proper, 8
Gold, Dr. (pseudonym), 175, 232; adjuvant therapy prescription, 201, 210, 213–14; chemotherapy, 36, 107; chemotherapy specialist, 56; medical oncologist, 50, 105–6; offer of help to patient, 206–9, 211; office visit with, 204–8; oncologist, 36; prescription after radiation, 201
Grace Hospital, 64, 69, 139
Gray, Dr. (pseudonym), 5, 10–12, 14–16, 66; attempts to contact, 33–5; cancer pronouncement, 12, 14, 18; gatekeepers of, 43, 47, 157, 170, 171; phone numbers from nurse, 49, 153; treatment plan, 24

Harvard, 20
healthcare providers, terms of endearment and, 69–70
health insurance: economy and, 113; Hong Kong, 27–8
HER2 positive, breast cancer cells, 21
Hippocrates, father of medicine, 12
Hippocratic oath, 211, 212
Hong Kong, 2, 14, 66, 73, 89, 146, 204, 215; April visit to see

Hong Kong (continued)
Father, 218–25; British colony
of, 7; Chinese society of, 90;
incidence of breast cancer,
25; medical treatment in, 15;
public and private healthcare
options, 27–8; public/private
healthcare system, 2; travel to,
25; treatment questions, 26–7;
treatments for patients, 116
Hong Kong Breast Cancer Foundation, 25
hydrocodone, 79
hypertension, blood pressure, 54
hypofractionation, 118, 187

illness, attitudes and, 103–4
immunotherapy, cancer treatment, 22, 23
incision: discussion on opening
of, 166–70; doctors blaming the
victim, 147–8, 184, 185; granulation, 195–6; packing procedure,
210; packing procedure for,
194–5; radiation and leaking
of, 139–44; scar for closed, 217;
searching for answers on leak,
143, 145–46; seeking assistance
for leaking fluid, 149–54
information technology, 214
insurance. See health insurance;
medical insurance
internal radiation, 118, 119
Islam, 233

Jansen, Dr. Chris (pseudonym),
anesthetist, 71–2
Japanese air raids, 7
Johns Hopkins, 20; Johns Hopkins
Hospital, 64
Jolie, Angelina, 66, 67, 107
juicing, vegetables, 99–100, 101–2

language: Chinese, 4, 9; English
pronunciation, 45; ignorance of
English, 121
letrozole, 201, 213, 219
Lewinsky, Monica, 151
life sentence, 2
live-in caregiver, Father's, 30–1,
61–2, 221
liver cancer, 21
Love, Susan, 20
lumpectomy, mastectomy or,
65–8, 81, 153, 193
lung cancer, 21
lymphedema, 139
lymph node: biopsy, 68; as
sentinel, 68

Makary, M., 169
mall walk, 130, 132–5
mammogram, 5, 10, 37; annual
screening, 22
mammography, 6–7
Marsh, Henry, 72, 120
mastectomy: choice of, 66; lumpectomy or, 65–8, 81, 153, 193
Mayo Clinic, 20
McEwan, Dr. (pseudonym), 231,
232; describing radiation and
treatment, 118–19; disappointment of patient in, 179–81;
education of, 117–18; focus of
killing cancer cells, 162–3; ignoring incision opening, 165–9,
174; on leaking incision, 142;
meetings after "resumed"
radiation, 165–9; oncologist,
36, 50; patient seeking help
for leaking incision, 149–55;
personal sharing of, 165; radiation, 36, 55, 56; recommending
surgeon appointment, 172;
scheduling radiation, 52, 53; as

"ultimate" professional, 168; visiting clinic for radiation, 129–30
medical appointments, coordinating, 39–47
medical associations, doctor treatment of patients, 231–2
medical bills: lacking resources for, 114; payment for, 108–13
medical fraud, guilt of oncologist Fata, 110–11, 160
medical insurance, 40–1, 42, 44, 46
medical knowledge, asymmetry in, 159
medical office, automatic answering device in, 33–5
medical protocol, breast cancer treatment, 52–3
medical science, breast cancer and, 80–1
metastasis, 13
MeToo movement, 180
Mexico, treatment costs in, 113
Mukerjhee, S., 20
muscle pain, 91

National Academy of Medicine, 38, 211
9/11 Museum in New York, 53
normalcy, 57; breast cancer robbing, 53
numbness in hands, 91

oncology 145; radiation, 158; surgical, 64
ONCOtype DX test, 107
opioid epidemic, 79

pain, post-surgery, 79–80
palliative radiation, spine, 13
parents, teaching of, 7–8
Parsons, Talcott, 158–9

pathetic fallacy, 87
"Pathology Report," 51
phone calls, support from friends, 93–5
plastic surgery technique, incision closure, 68–9
post-surgery: fatigue, 80, 81–4; pain, 79–80
preparatory doctor, surgery, 72–5
private healthcare system, advocates of, 114
Professional Dominance (Freidson), 38
progesterone receptor positive, breast cancer cells, 21
prostate cancer, Father's, 2, 3, 5, 13, 61
psychology books, on disease diagnosis, 59
public healthcare system, 2, 3; Hong Kong, 116

quacks, taking advantage of sick, 192
questioning superiors, cultural training, 49

radiation: arm stretches, 139; breathing for treatments, 125–6; burning skin on breast, 141; cancer treatment, 22–3; clinic, 117; complications in, 86–7; concerns of over-radiation, 170; control room for, 124–7; description of treatment, 118–19; experiences of others, 55–6; fallouts from, 55; incision closure before, 146; leaking incision, 139–44; medical protocol for, 52, 53; number of sessions, 119–20; pictures of breast for medical physicist and dosimetrist,

radiation *(continued)*
122–3; preparation of, 119, 121, 127; reluctance in returning to, 159–61; Ruby and John operating radiation bunker, 124–6; Ruby obtaining antibiotic ointment for incision, 172–3; scheduling of, 50, 230; seeking advice for breast cancer, 146–8; seeking help for leaking incision, 149–55; shopping aerobics and, 137–8; souvenir mug, 173; surgery and, 68; tattooing for, 122
relationship, communication changes, 57–8
"remission": term, 25–6; term "in remission," 23, 26
reverse ageism, 75

SARS origin, 97
Saving Graces (Edwards), 90
Second World War, 7, 220
seroma, radiation and, 142
sexual harassment, 180
Shield, Dr. (pseudonym), 232; absence of bra and, 183–5, 187, 197; compliment on patient's toughness, 197–9; examination of incision, 182–8; on granulations, 195–6; lumpectomy or mastectomy, 65–8; office appointment with, 64–5; packing procedure, 194–5; post-surgery 77; presentation of, 65; referral for, 52; seeking appointment for incision, 175, 177–9; surgeon, 50; surgery, 56, 76, 116; treating opened incision, 189–94; version of patient-centeredness 194; website and reviews of, 63–4
shingles, 26

shopping, 133–7; "shopping aerobics," 137–8
Sino-British Joint Declaration (1984), 89
sleep, fatigue and, 84–5
social life, equity in, 180–1
sonogram, 6; breast, 8–9
souvenir mug, radiation office, 173
specialists, treatment requiring, 35–6
spine, cancer spreading to, 13
staging, breast cancer, 21, 24
Stanford, 20
Starr, Paul, 158
stomach cancer, 91
stress, damage to body, 209
stroke, 30
support group, 39; experiences of doctors sharing information, 202; medical care costs, 115–16; solace from, 91–3; treatment options, 113–14
surgery 4; anesthetist, 71–2; cancer treatment, 22; checking in for, 69–71; diagnostic radiologist, 74–6; experiences of others, 55–6; lumpectomy or mastectomy choice, 65–8; operating room, 76; picking a treatment, 65–6; plans before, 85; post-op room, 76–7; preparatory doctor, 72–5; scheduling, 50; waiting for, 55; *see also* post-surgery
surgical oncology, 64
systemic radiation, 118, 119

target therapy, cancer treatment, 22, 23
throat cancer, 92, 93
treatments, cancer patients seeking, 109–10
tumor(s), 17; biopsy, 9–10; breast, 6; size of, 66

ultrasound, 6, 10
Unaccountable (Makary), 169
United Airline Flight 93 53
United Kingdom, 20
United States, 20; breast cancer,
    21; insurance premiums, 115;
    National Academy of Medicine,
    38; treatment costs, 116

Valley of Death, 161
Victor (husband), 11–12, 16, 24,
    29, 30, 31, 57, 60, 62, 71, 80, 83,
    131–2, 140–1, 171–2, 213; call to
    Dr. Shield's office, 178–9

white blood cell counts,
    chemotherapy, 153
woman doctor, disappointment in
    Dr. McEwan, 179–81

X-ray: breast cancer, 118, 119;
    mammography, 6; radiation,
    118, 119; strength of, 143–4;
    tumor, 122, 123, 126–7, 143, 161

Yale, 20
yin and yang, 96
Youde Hospital, 2; urology
    department, 2